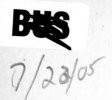

7/22/05

The Expert Guide
to Beating Heart Disease

The Expert Guide
to Beating Heart Disease

WHAT YOU ABSOLUTELY MUST KNOW

HARLAN M. KRUMHOLZ, M.D.

A HarperResource Book

An Imprint of HarperCollins*Publishers*

FIRST EDITION
Designed by Fritz Metsch

Library of Congress Cataloging-in-Publication Data
Krumholz, Harlan M.
   The expert guide to beating heart disease : what you absolutely must know / Harlan
   M. Krumholz.
      p. cm.
   Includes bibliographical references and index.
   ISBN: 0-06-057834-3
      1. Heart—Diseases—Popular works. I. Title.
RC672.K78 2005
616.1'2—dc22   2004054234

05 06 07 08 09 WBC/RRD 10 9 8 7 6 5 4 3 2 1

CONTENTS

In *The Expert Guide to Beating Heart Disease*, respected cardiologist Harlan Krumholz has built the bridge between the lifesaving research results of our laboratories and the ultimate beneficiaries of the research, the patients. Our medical journals are replete with bench research and clinical trials whose results contain remarkable insights that have changed our thinking about the prevention, diagnosis, and treatment of heart disease, yet the sluggish way that this critically important information often makes its way into practice limits its usefulness. A neglected way to speed the process of incorporating new advances is to rely on the public's great interest in matters related to their own health, and that is just what Dr. Krumholz has accomplished.

People want to be in a position to benefit from the latest medical knowledge—and yet not be a victim of the hype and unfounded claims of so-called miracle cures. Patients must be willing to get involved, to believe that it is their business to know about the options for tests, for treatments, and for preventive measures that will help them avoid the serious consequences of disease. Patients must be their own advocates and participate actively in decisions with their doctors and nurses. Good doctors welcome such involvement. Nobody needs a medical degree to learn about what is best for them; what they need is the right attitude and accurate, simple-to-understand information.

The Expert Guide to Beating Heart Disease provides a way for patients with heart disease to ensure that they are giving themselves the best chance for good health and health care. Knowledge is the best tool for any patient to guarantee that they are getting the best care. What they need is a source that is credible, trustworthy, and understandable, and Dr. Krumholz, an international expert on cardiovascular disease—and a leader in improving the quality of health care—provides it. Dr. Krumholz has distilled the most important information that every patient with heart disease (or a potential for developing it) should know.

His guide should be read by every patient with heart disease and those who want to protect themselves against the ravages of a disease that kills and disables so many.

Jerome P. Kassirer, M.D.
Distinguished Professor, Tufts University School of Medicine
Editor-in-Chief Emeritus, *New England Journal of Medicine*

A Letter from the Doctor

If you're reading this book, it's likely that you or someone you care about has heart disease. Heart disease is the leading cause of death in America and most other industrialized nations. This condition is usually caused by fatty deposits accumulating and building up inside the arteries that supply nutrients and oxygen-rich blood to your heart. When that blood flow becomes restricted by the narrowing of the arteries, your heart starts sending distress signals. The first sign of trouble may be shortness of breath when climbing stairs. Or sudden chest pain, called *angina*. Or a heart attack.

Whatever the first sign is, heart disease changes your life forever. It is chronic; that is, we don't yet know how to cure it. Of the millions of Americans with heart disease today, one million will have a heart attack this year and more than half of them will die as a result. That's the bad news.

The good news is that recent scientific breakthroughs have made it possible to control and in some cases even reverse your heart disease. Today, as a result of these advances, more people are surviving heart disease and heart attacks than ever before. Ironically, this also means that more people now have to live with heart disease every day. What you need most now is information: trustworthy, scientifically accurate, and easily understandable information about what you can do to give yourself the best chance of taking charge of your heart disease.

You'd think that would be easy, given all the information that's currently available. But it's not. Sure, there are lots of books, mag-

azine and newspaper articles, TV reports, pamphlets, advertise-
ments, and websites offering information on heart disease. But it's
nearly impossible to sort out what information is reliable—that is,
grounded in the best science and unbiased—and what is not.

Fortunately, there *are* highly regarded sources of thoroughly
credible information on the best strategies for treating your heart
disease. The sources with some of the most helpful information for
people with heart disease are guidelines published by the American
Heart Association and the American College of Cardiology. Com-
piled by the best heart specialists in the country and updated regularly, their recommendations provide the very best information
available on various aspects of heart disease.

The problem is that these guidelines are written for doctors.

That's where this book comes in. *The Expert Guide to Beating
Heart Disease* translates these expert guidelines and the best evidence about heart disease into plain English. This book gives you
the key strategies that researchers have found work best. It equips
you to monitor and enhance your own care. It also explains new,
unproven, and even controversial treatments so you know exactly
where the research on these treatments stands.

There's another reason why this book is important for you. Research into the treatment of heart disease patients has shown time
and again that there is a substantial gap between what scientists
and expert cardiologists know about treating heart disease and
how much of that knowledge is put to work for patients. In truth,
the quality of care heart disease patients receive varies from place
to place and from doctor to doctor. This book will help you ensure
that you're getting the best, most effective treatment possible. It
will also make it easier to understand the relative importance of
each treatment your doctor recommends. This book encourages
you to be engaged actively in your own treatment plan. After all,
no one has a greater stake in the outcome of your treatment than
you. With this book, you'll have the tools to make informed
choices so you can beat heart disease.

My intention is to place the best medical knowledge on heart disease directly in your hands so you can take charge of your heart disease—and your health.

Harlan M. Krumholz, M.D., S.M.
Professor of Medicine (Cardiology)
Yale University School of Medicine

ACKNOWLEDGMENTS

I owe a special thanks to the John A. Hartford Foundation and Mr. William T. Comfort, Jr. They provided the impetus for this book and the financial support that sustained it. This effort would not have been possible without them.

I also owe a great debt to the many people who contributed to this book. In particular, Dr. Susan Cheng, who worked with me as a research assistant, helped forge the vision for this book and contributed substantially to its content. Susan has a remarkable commitment to improving patient care, and I was fortunate to have had the opportunity to work with her. The book also benefited from the valuable input of patients, friends, and colleagues too numerous to list here. In particular, I am grateful to Maureen O'Connor, R.N., and a special group of cardiac rehabilitation participants who generously contributed their time to provide feedback. My goal was to present medical information in a manner that would be easily understood by the reader. William E. Nothdurft made important contributions in this respect, helping to improve the communication of the scientific content. This publication would not have been possible without the outstanding contributions of my agent, Jennifer Joel, and my editor, Toni Sciarra. I also owe special thanks to Maria Johnson, my administrative assistant, who served as an astute reader and editor. Dr. Jerry Kassirer was a constant source of support, and kindly agreed to pen a foreword for the book. Most importantly, I am grateful for the support of my family, who were so critical to the successful completion of this project.

How to Use This Book

This book is organized so you can find the heart disease treatment information you need easily and quickly.

Chapter 1, "Understanding Heart Disease," explains, clearly and concisely, what you need to know about your disease. We explore what heart disease is, how it's caused, the risk factors that cause it to occur in some people but not others, its most common symptoms, and how doctors investigate those symptoms.

Chapter 2, "Seven Key Strategies for Taking Charge of Heart Disease," contains some of the most important information in this book. It describes seven *key strategies* for treating heart disease. Each of these strategies is based on the official expert guidelines published for doctors, nurses, and other health care professionals by the American Heart Association (AHA) and the American College of Cardiology (ACC), among others. The scientific evidence behind the strongest recommendations in these guidelines is very solid. These recommendations represent the proven strategies and treatments that the best doctors and scientists in cardiology agree really work. Everyone with heart disease should know them. Now you can. By using these strategies as a checklist, you can make sure you're getting the best care available. You'll have the tools you need to help yourself get better.

Chapter 3, "Beyond the Key Strategies," explores other important components of your heart disease treatment program. We examine treatment alternatives that are not strongly recommended by the guidelines, mainly because the medical evidence on how well they work is not yet conclusive. Indeed, some of these treatments have no demonstrated benefits at all—and may even be harmful. But that doesn't mean you shouldn't know about them. Quite the contrary; the more you know about the strengths and weaknesses of different kinds of treatments, the easier it will be for you to choose wisely among them. If you are willing to bet on the value of treatment alternatives that haven't yet been proven effective, you should know about how strongly the available research evidence supports those treatments.

Chapter 4, "Research and Emerging Therapies," explores what's on the medical horizon for treating heart disease, specifically a half-dozen or so therapies that are currently being studied and may be recommended in the not-too-distant future.

Chapter 5, "Staying Well and Prepared," concludes with information you'll want to know while you're on the road to recovery. It shows you how to monitor the health of your heart, highlights other health risks you'll want to guard against, and suggests ways to make the most of your visits to the doctor.

Finally, at the end of the book, you'll find helpful Appendices. This portion of the book is a toolbox of sorts that includes information on tests and procedures you may undergo during the treatment and monitoring of your heart disease, as well as progress logs and checklists. It also contains information about possible problems with certain combinations of drugs. A Resources section guides you to sources of more detailed information on many of the topics summarized in this book. A Glossary provides quick definitions of medical terms. A References section lists the sources of every medical study and research result mentioned in the book. And there is a comprehensive Index so you can find what you're looking for in this book easily and quickly.

It's my hope that you won't just read through this book once, but will keep it handy as a resource you can turn to over and over as you begin the journey of overcoming heart disease.

Throughout the book I describe many approaches that are used to prevent heart disease. To give you a sense of the importance of each approach, I have marked each section with one of the symbols shown below. These symbols can help you quickly identify which treatments are the most strongly supported by experts and evidence and which ones are not. In Appendix A, you'll find a Quick Guide to Heart Disease Treatments that uses this symbol-grading system to show the range of treatments—from the most to the least reputable.

Grading of Treatments Commonly Used to Fight Heart Disease	
★★★	**Proven benefit.** Three stars indicate that a large amount of scientific research supports the use of this treatment. If you are not taking advantage of this treatment, then you should know why not.
★★	**Probable benefit.** Two stars indicate that there is some disagreement about the effect of this treatment, but that it may benefit you.
★	**Possible benefit.** One star means that the treatment is promising, but there is not yet enough evidence to strongly recommend it.
⑦	**Unclear effect.** This symbol means there is not yet enough research to indicate whether the treatment has any effect–good or bad–on the heart.
⊘	**No effect.** This symbol means that research shows that the treatment has no effect on the heart.
ⓘ	**Harmful.** This symbol means that research shows that the treatment is harmful.

CHAPTER 1

Understanding Heart Disease

The human heart is an astonishing organ. A muscle only about the size of your fist, it sits just to the left of the center of your chest contracting and relaxing to pump blood—roughly five liters of it a minute—throughout your body. It is an involuntary muscle. Unlike, for example, the muscles in your arm that you flex voluntarily when you lift something, your heart needs no instruction. It operates independently and continuously, day and night, week in, week out, year after year. When it stops, life stops.

What Is Heart Disease?

The heart is tough, but it's not invulnerable and it can be afflicted by a variety of diseases. But what's commonly called heart disease (though, more accurately known as "coronary artery disease") is, interestingly enough, not a disease of the heart at all. At least not directly. It's a disease of the large arteries outside the heart that supply the smaller vessels that feed the heart muscle with blood rich in nutrients and oxygen that the heart needs to keep working. Other vessels carry away the waste products produced by the heart in the course of its work. Coronary arteries, the large arteries carrying blood to the heart muscle, are like the huge pipes that carry water from a reservoir to a big city, to be distributed to streets, individual houses, and then specific faucets before being carried away again through drains. If something happens to those big pipes that blocks the flow of vital water to the city, the city shuts down in no time at all. Your heart needs an open system of pipes to maintain an unabated flow of blood all the time.

When the heart works harder, such as during exertion or stress, it needs even more blood flow. It gets this greater flow because, unlike water pipes, the blood vessels can dilate, or open larger, when the need arises. When something impedes that flow, it causes immediate problems for the heart muscle, which becomes starved of oxygen and nutrients.

With heart disease, the "something" that restricts the flow is an accumulation of fatty deposits—including cholesterol—that form thick "plaques" on the interior walls of the coronary arteries, a process that can slow the flow of blood to the heart. This condition, called *atherosclerosis*, occurs gradually and may go unnoticed for years.

What Are the Symptoms of Heart Disease?

When atherosclerosis is advanced, the flow of blood can be reduced enough that when the heart is asked to work harder than usual—for example, when you're exercising or climbing stairs, or simply digesting a heavy meal—it can't get the blood flow that it needs.

Typically, the heart signals that it's struggling by producing a feeling of chest discomfort, a condition that doctors call *angina*. Angina can take many forms; the sensations can include weakness, heaviness, pressure, tightness, and even pain in the middle of the chest. People with angina may also feel this discomfort at some distance from the heart—in the arms, abdomen, back, neck, and lower jaw, for example. Angina is simply the heart's way of saying there is a mismatch between the oxygen-rich blood flow it needs and what is actually arriving for its use. Usually, if you have this symptom, the discomfort goes away when you stop whatever activity is causing your heart to work harder than usual (or, if you've already been diagnosed with angina, when you take medication, such as nitroglycerin tablets or spray). You should also know that not everyone has this feeling when there is a problem with blood flow to the heart, but it usually is an important signal when it occurs.

If you experience any symptoms in the checklist below, you should let your doctor know because they could be indications of heart disease. These symptoms are not always caused by heart disease; they may be harmless or due to other medical conditions. But if you already have heart disease, these symptoms are enough to indicate a potential heart problem and reason enough for you to check with your doctor, especially if these symptoms are new.

- **DISCOMFORT IN YOUR CHEST** that comes on during physical exertion or emotional stress; it may spread to your arms, neck, lower jaw, face, back, or stomach. If this discomfort is from your heart, it is called *angina*.

- **UNUSUAL BREATHLESSNESS** when doing light activity or when you are at rest can be a symptom of heart disease. Breathlessness that comes on suddenly may be an important warning sign.

- **PALPITATION** is the term used to describe the condition in which you feel your heart beat faster or more forcefully than usual, or in an irregular pattern. Palpitations may be a symptom of heart disease, especially if they last for a few hours, if they come and go over several days, or if they cause chest pain, breathlessness, or dizziness.

- **FAINTING** (or the sensation that you are about to faint) can be caused by inadequate oxygen reaching the brain, which may be due to heart disease.

- **SWELLING** or fluid retention (also known as *edema*) is fluid buildup in your tissues. This usually happens around the ankles, legs, lungs, and abdomen. Swelling of the legs can be perfectly normal for some people after working many hours on their feet. However, it can also be a sign that the heart is not pumping efficiently.

- **FATIGUE** has many causes, but it's worth seeing the doctor if you feel unusually tired, especially if it is combined with other suspicious symptoms noted above.

Sometimes, however, the danger signal from the heart is more dramatic. Atherosclerosis causes plaques to accumulate in the coronary arteries. These plaques are lumps and bumps within the coronary arteries that can contain cholesterol, white blood cells, and other substances. Sometimes they grow to block the arteries and sometimes they are small and do not affect the blood flow. A cap forms on top of the plaque to keep the contents from seeping into the bloodstream. These plaques can be quiescent and not cause a problem. Occasionally, however, the cap on a plaque can rupture (and this can happen on a big or small plaque), exposing its contents to the bloodstream. When this happens, the contents of the plaque are mixed with the blood and can cause formation of a blood clot. If the blood clot blocks an important artery supplying blood to the heart, heart muscle can be suddenly deprived of vital oxygen and nutrients. At this point, every minute counts because heart muscle cannot survive long without receiving fresh blood. Within a relatively short period the damage to the heart can be severe and permanent. This event is what doctors call a *myocardial infarction.*

Everyone else calls it a heart attack.

The symptoms of a heart attack are often similar to those of angina, but much worse and more persistent. The classic description of a heart attack is a "crushing chest pain" that does not go away, even after resting or taking angina medication. Other symptoms, which sometimes can even occur without chest pain, can include sweating, nausea, light-headedness, and breathlessness. These symptoms are often confused with those caused by other, much less serious conditions.

Here's the important thing to keep in mind: Don't take chances. If you experience symptoms that may represent a heart attack, you should call an ambulance immediately and be brought to an emergency department; your survival may depend upon it. It is natural to feel reluctant to ask for help, and for many people it is embarrassing to call an ambulance. Also, heart attacks often do not start like they do in the movies, with crushing pain that causes you to clutch your chest. Uncertainty is quite common, but you should not wait to see whether your condition gets worse. This is the time to call 911.

As a general rule, doctors recommend that angina-like discomfort that occurs without exertion or persists for more than ten minutes should be treated as a sign of a possible heart attack, even if more dramatic symptoms do not develop. The National Heart, Lung, and Blood Institute of the National Institutes of Health recommends that people should not wait more than five minutes before calling 911. Why the rush? Treatment, particularly in the first hour, can make an enormous difference in improving a person's chance of survival. Unfortunately, most people experiencing a heart attack wait much longer to seek help. According to experts, most people wait two or more hours before obtaining medical attention.

How Is Heart Disease Diagnosed?

Based upon a physical examination and your answers to questions about your symptoms, medical history, and habits (such as smoking) that are known to put you at risk, your doctor may suspect heart disease. The next step is to conduct tests to determine the presence, type, severity, and cause of the heart condition. (You can learn more about these tests by turning to the Tests and Medical Procedures section in the Appendices of this book.) Tests used to investigate heart disease and its consequences may include:

- Blood and urine tests;

- Electrocardiogram (also called an ECG or EKG), which shows information about the heart based on its electrical activity;

- Chest X-ray;

- Echocardiogram, which uses sound waves to view the heart;

- Stress tests, in which you either walk on a treadmill or receive a medication and the effects on your heart are examined by your symptoms, an ECG, and sometimes also by pictures of the heart (also called an imaging test, which is conducted by an echocardiogram or a scan of your heart after the injection of a radioactive substance that can be detected by special cameras);

- Cardiac catheterization (also called an angiogram), in which a special X-ray procedure is done to look at the heart's blood supply;

- CT scan, which is used to look for calcium in the arteries, a tell-tale sign of coronary artery disease; and

- MRI, a new test that is not yet commonly used in clinical practice, which provides pictures of the heart and information about narrowing of the arteries.

Why Me? Who Gets Heart Disease?

Coronary heart disease is the world's most common heart ailment. In the United States alone, more than 12 million people have the disease and another 650,000 people are diagnosed with it each year. Heart disease affects women and men, both old and young, and is the leading cause of death and disability among adults.

Over the years, researchers have demonstrated conclusively that some people are more susceptible to heart disease than others. The most famous of these studies, the Framingham Heart Study, tracked the health of more than 5,000 residents of Framingham, Massachusetts, to find out what factors contributed to heart disease. In time, the family members and children of these original subjects also became part of the study. Now the grandchildren are being invited to participate.

Over the course of half a century, the researchers have identified a number of characteristics, commonly called risk factors, that are associated with heart disease. Some of these risk factors can't be changed—and doctors call them "non-modifiable" risk factors. Age is one. No matter who you are, the older you are, the higher your risk of heart disease. Your family history is another. If others in your family have had heart disease, your own risk of the disease is higher than someone with no heart disease in his or her family.

Non-Modifiable Risk Factors

- **AGE:** you are a man over 45 or a woman over 55

- **FAMILY HISTORY:** your father or brother had a heart attack before 55, or your mother or sister before 65

But many risk factors involve conditions or ways of living that you can do something about—and doctors call these "modifiable."

Modifiable Risk Factors

- **HIGH BLOOD PRESSURE:** your blood pressure is greater than 140/90 mmHg (or 130/80 mmHg if you have diabetes or kidney dysfunction) and/or you've been told your blood pressure is too high

- **HIGH BLOOD CHOLESTEROL:** if you have heart disease, your total cholesterol level is 200 mg/dL or higher or your LDL ("bad cholesterol") is 100 mg/dL or higher (70 mg/dL or higher for high-risk individuals) or your HDL ("good cholesterol") is less than 40 mg/dL

- **DIABETES OR HIGH BLOOD SUGAR:** you have diagnosed diabetes or a fasting blood sugar level of 126 mg/dL or higher

- **OVERWEIGHT:** you have a body mass index (BMI) score of 25 or more (see page 64 for chart)

- **PHYSICAL INACTIVITY:** you exercise (or exert yourself) less than 30 minutes per day

- **SMOKING:** you are a smoker

These factors don't just increase your risk for heart disease; if you already have heart disease, they increase your risk of future heart problems.

Taking Charge: Seven Key Strategies

When it comes to beating heart disease, information is important but action is critical. This book spells out the very best medical knowledge on heart disease treatment available today, knowledge that can help you get the best possible care available and protect you from future heart problems. But information alone won't cure you of heart disease. What will make the difference between illness and health is your own active involvement in your treatment.

Here's a good example: national surveys have revealed that many people with high blood pressure are never even identified as having this life-threatening condition. Of those who are identified, many are not treated. Of those who are treated, many do not receive the correct treatment to ensure that their blood pressure is properly controlled, including being advised about the critical importance of taking their medication regularly. Because high blood pressure causes no obvious symptoms (until it gets extremely high or causes complications) many people have no sense of the seriousness of their condition and do not take their medications. The result? Every year there are hundreds, even thousands, of preventable heart attacks and strokes related to high blood pressure. By contrast, patients who are involved actively in their own care, who understand the importance of controlling their blood pressure, and who work with their doctor to do so, often can avoid this result.

There's another reason for taking charge of your own heart disease. Because there is no "typical" heart disease patient, your illness is different from any other heart disease patient's, and your experience of the illness and the treatments that are best for you may differ as well. Since every patient is different, doctors need to customize the treatment options available to meet the individual needs and preferences of each patient. The more you know about your heart disease and the options available to you, the more likely it is that you'll succeed in working with your physician to develop a plan that is best for you and most likely to lead to the results you want.

This means you have a shared responsibility for your care. It is true that doctors undergo years of training so they can diagnose, treat, and manage diseases. But when it comes to your own health, nobody knows your needs and preferences better than you do. Since much of what will need to be done for you to recover from heart disease must be done *by you*, your doctor's role over the long term is to provide guidance—but *you* are the key. Good doctors welcome and encourage their patients to participate in their own care—for the simple reason that it yields better health results.

Only about sixty years ago, the most powerful man in the world, President Franklin Delano Roosevelt, died from a stroke because his doctors had no effective medicine to treat his high blood pressure. They were powerless to reduce his risk as his heart disease worsened. Today, we can—or, more accurately, *you* can. The good news is that scientific advances made during the last fifty years have improved the outlook for heart disease patients dramatically. Not only do we know what puts people at risk for heart disease, we also have evidence that certain strategies will lower these risks.

How strong is this evidence? So strong that it represents the top strategies recommended for doctors, nurses, and other health professionals by the American Heart Association, the American College of Cardiology, and other groups.

Not surprisingly, perhaps, these strategies aim squarely at those risk factors that are modifiable—that is, those you can do something about:

The Key Strategies

1. Control your blood pressure

2. Manage your cholesterol

3. Exercise

4. Control your weight

5. Watch your blood sugars

6. Quit smoking

7. Take the right medications

In the next part of this book, we explore each of these strategies in detail.

A PATIENT'S VIEW:
TAKING CHARGE AT ANY AGE

I was born in the Northeast and for twenty-five years I owned and ran a business. Almost twenty years ago I found out the hard way that I had heart disease. I was vacationing with my wife, and we went out for a big meal—I remember that we had lots of good food and beer that night. Before going to bed I developed crushing chest pain and rushed to a hospital where, after a couple of hours, they told me that I had indigestion. They gave me an antacid and sent me back to the hotel.

When I returned home I called my doctor, who sent me for a stress test. Well, I flunked and was promptly sent for an angiogram. After the test the doctor sat me down and told me that I was a walking time bomb. He said that if we didn't do something right away that I'd look good in a box. That really scared me. Honestly, that was just what he told me. He then said that I needed bypass.

I didn't even know what he was talking about. I asked him if he meant open heart surgery. He nodded. A day later I had triple bypass.

I still can barely believe that happened to me. I was not overweight. My cholesterol and blood pressure were under control. I didn't exercise much or pay much attention to my diet, but I didn't think it mattered much.

The recovery was lousy and it was a month or more before I started feeling better. I definitely realized that life was wonderful and from that moment my whole life changed. Everything changed. I went to cardiac rehabilitation and got hooked on exercise. I have worked out for about two hours a day for the past twenty years. A half hour on the treadmill. Another fifteen minutes on the bicycle. Other exercises, too. And then weights three times a week. Five days a week I am up at five and exercising by six. On the weekends I do sleep in, but I still get in my exercise. Also, I changed my diet—now I pay close attention to what I eat.

I also pay attention to my medications. I keep careful records of my medications—I carry a card with me that lists them. I never miss a dose. And my wife makes sure of that.

I learned about what was good for my heart and stick to it. And I made good friends. All of us had setbacks with our hearts but are now stronger than ever.

I recently turned ninety. I never felt so good.

.—Howard

CHAPTER 2

Seven Key Strategies for
Taking Charge of Heart Disease

Strategy #1:
★★★ Take Charge of Your Blood Pressure

Place a finger just below the bone that protrudes on the inside of your wrist, just below your thumb. That rhythmic pulsing you feel is, quite literally, the surge of blood propelled from your heart. Your heart beats roughly 100,000 times a day. Each time it does, it pushes blood into your blood vessels and, through them, to all the cells of your body. Blood pressure is a measure of the force of blood moving with each heartbeat *and* of the force those elastic vessel walls exert on the blood flowing through them. The first person ever to measure these forces was Stephen Hale, an eighteenth-century English clergyman who was also a leading botanist, chemist, physiologist, and inventor. Having done pioneering work on the physiology of plants, Hale moved on to animals. In 1733, he used a nine-foot-long vertical glass tube to measure the pressure exerted by blood in blood vessels. His "patient" was a horse.

Blood pressure keeps nutrients and oxygen moving to the body's cells in the vast recycling system that is your circulation. It's called "circulatory" because the entire system is a constantly repeating cycle. You may have noticed over the years when you've cut yourself that sometimes the blood that escapes is bright red and sometimes it's dark. The bright red blood is full of freshly oxygenated cells and loaded with nutrients. The dark red blood is, in effect, the "used-up" blood that's circling its way back to exchange carbon dioxide for oxygen. The squeezing of the heart moves the blood around and creates the pressure. The pressure must be sufficient to overcome the force of gravity and reach your head when you stand.

Quite simply, blood pressure is what keeps you alive. But if it's too high, it can also harm you.

The Silent Killer

When blood pressure is too high for too long it can scar, stiffen, and narrow the insides of your blood vessels, forcing your heart to work harder than it should. Like any other muscle, working harder can cause the heart to thicken. Unlike other muscles, however, thickening can make the heart weaker, not stronger. A bulging bicep may be a good thing; a heart that is too muscular is not. At the same time, narrower and less elastic blood vessels create conditions in which blood clots can become stuck and block blood flow. In time, faced with these challenges, the heart can begin to wear out, sending less blood to your body with each beat than your body really needs, a condition known as "heart failure." But you may never be aware that any of this is happening.

High blood pressure—also called *hypertension*—is known as "the silent killer" because it generally has no outward symptoms. It can sometimes cause headaches or dizziness or fatigue, but these symptoms are vague and often attributed to other, less serious causes. All too often, the first "symptom" is a heart attack or stroke. The higher your blood pressure, the higher your risk.

More than 65 million Americans have high blood pressure—that's one out of every three adults. For every ten people who have high blood pressure, three have no idea they have it. Of those who know they have hypertension, some 15 percent (about 1 in 6) are not being treated. Of those who are being treated, almost one half aren't being treated regularly enough or well enough to bring their blood pressure down to safe levels.

Your chances of having high blood pressure increase as you age. Researchers from the Framingham Heart Study recently found that Americans who are fifty-five years old and older have a 90 percent chance of developing high blood pressure during their lifetime.

Getting Your Blood Pressure Tested

The only way high blood pressure can be detected is by a blood pressure measurement. For this reason, and because health professionals now understand the direct link between high blood pressure and other diseases, one of the first things a nurse or doctor will do when you have an appointment—for almost any reason—is check your blood pressure.

Blood pressure is measured in much the same way as atmospheric pressure is assessed with a weather barometer: in units of millimeters of mercury (or, mmHg). The pressurized cuff placed around your arm effectively determines the point at which your existing blood pressure is overcome by the pressure in the cuff.

Unlike other measures, like your temperature, however, blood pressure gives you two numbers, not one. The person taking your blood pressure will document the results as the first number "over" the second number. The first number in a blood pressure reading is your *systolic* blood pressure. That's the pressure produced in your blood vessels during each contraction, or "beat" of your heart. The second number is your *diastolic* blood pressure. It's the pressure inside your arteries when your heart relaxes between beats.

Unlike temperature, there is no one number that is considered normal for blood pressure. Higher blood pressure is generally associated with higher risk, but there is no number that is considered just right. In general, lower blood pressure is better as long as you do not have any side effects, such as light-headedness.

The measurement of blood pressure is not always consistent. Blood pressure varies from individual to individual and, for that matter, at different times of the day, depending upon the demands and stresses placed upon your heart. If you're caught in traffic and rush in late for your doctor's appointment, for example, the chances are you'll have a higher blood pressure reading than if you had a leisurely walk. Because of this variation, national experts have made some suggestions about what you should do before your blood pressure reading. National guidelines suggest that patients should follow these steps:

- Avoid smoking or drinking caffeine 30 minutes before having your blood pressure measured.

- Rest for 5 minutes before the measurement is taken.

- When your blood pressure is being measured, be seated with your feet flat on the floor, back and arm supported, arm at heart level; after the first measurement, rest for 2 minutes before the second measurement; a second measurement is recommended to confirm the first. If the first two readings differ by more than 5 mmHg, then a third measurement is recommended.

What Do the Guidelines Recommend?

While there is no "normal" blood pressure reading, doctors now know enough about the relationship between blood pressure and heart disease—and other diseases as well—to know which range of blood pressure readings is safer and which is more dangerous. Ideally, your doctor would like to see your blood pressure levels lower than 120 over 80 (120/80), though higher levels are still considered within a lower risk range.

The most authoritative recommendations about blood pressure derive from the National Institutes of Health's Joint National Committee on Prevention, Detection, Evaluation, and Treatment of High Blood Pressure, which represents the opinion of the

How High Is My Blood Pressure?			
Category	Systolic		Diastolic
Normal	<120	and	<80
Pre-Hypertension	120–139	and	80–89
Hypertension			
Stage 1	140–159	or	90–99
Stage 2	≥160	or	≥100

nation's experts. These guidelines recommend that everyone's blood pressure should be lower than 140/90, because just above that level, known as Stage 1 hypertension, there is agreement that your risk is higher than it should be. As a result, the target blood pressure for most people is 140/90 or lower. For every 20 mmHg increase in a person's systolic blood pressure or every 10 mmHg increase in a person's diastolic blood pressure, the risk for heart problems or stroke doubles.

While the Joint National Committee urges most people to keep their blood pressure below 140/90, they set even lower targets for patients with a higher risk of health problems due to hypertension. If you have diabetes or kidney failure (a condition where the kidneys are unable to filter the body's blood as effectively as needed), the committee recommends that your blood pressure should be below 130/80.

If you have heart disease, there's a good chance you have high blood pressure as well; the two often go hand in hand. Taking charge of your heart disease means taking charge of your hypertension, because reducing your high blood pressure can reduce your risk for more severe heart trouble by 20 percent. Many studies have shown that lowering high blood pressure also reduces your risk for stroke by at least 30 percent and your risk of dying from a heart problem or stroke by at least 20 percent.

If, as a result of several measurements, your blood pressure is consistently above the target levels, your doctor will probably recommend other tests, including urinalysis (urine test), a blood count, a blood chemistry analysis (testing levels of potassium, sodium, creatinine [an indicator for kidney disease], and glucose [blood sugar]), a check of your cholesterol levels, and perhaps an electrocardiogram. Each of these tests tells the doctor something about your risk, the possible causes of your hypertension (including some rare causes that may require special treatment), their consequences, and your potential risk for further disease.

Doctors often classify hypertension into two forms. The first and most common type is known as *essential hypertension*. The cause is not known and is under active investigation, though it may be associated with narrowed and stiff arteries. The second, and more unusual, form is called *secondary hypertension*. As its name suggests, in this case the hypertension is actually secondary to some other condition altogether, such as kidney disease, and is best addressed by treating that other underlying disease. Your doctor may suspect secondary hypertension if your blood pressure fluctuates significantly, is extremely high, doesn't respond to hypertension medications, or has been present since you were young. For most people, no other cause is ever found and they are left with a diagnosis of essential hypertension.

Whatever its form, hypertension is dangerous and you may well want to keep track of your blood pressure more frequently than just when you see your doctor. There are many options for people who want to keep close watch on their blood pressure. You may be able to have your blood pressure checked free at your local drugstore or supermarket. But you may also wish to purchase a blood pressure monitoring device you can use at home. If you do, you should know that home monitoring devices can vary in quality. So be sure to bring your device along when you visit your doctor to compare your readings with your doctor's device on a regular basis.

Lowering Blood Pressure with Lifestyle Changes

The good news about high blood pressure is that it's readily treatable—and much of the treatment is within your own control. The expert recommendations for what you should do to treat your hypertension depend upon your blood pressure readings.

If you have heart disease and your blood pressure is in what's called the "high-normal" range (systolic 130–139; diastolic 85–89), you may not require medication. Your doctor will probably recommend that you first try to reduce your blood pressure by changing your lifestyle. It's easy to dismiss this advice, but there is excellent evidence that this approach can make a big difference. In addition, if you can avoid medications, you can avoid their cost and potential adverse effects. Before going on medication, you should give a drug-free strategy a chance. This "lifestyle approach" to treatment may involve five steps:

1. **LOSE YOUR EXTRA WEIGHT.** Studies show that if you are overweight, losing even 10 pounds will lower your blood pressure. And if you do need to take blood pressure–lowering medications, cutting your weight will increase their effectiveness. (See the DASH Diet on pages 26–30.)

2. **LIMIT YOUR ALCOHOL** to no more than 24 ounces of beer, 20 ounces of wine, or 2 ounces of whiskey per day. Excess alcohol can not only cause hypertension and stroke, but can also interfere with blood pressure–lowering medications.

3. **EXERCISE** 30 to 45 minutes per day, most days of the week. People who are inactive have a 20 to 50 percent higher chance of developing hypertension. If you do have hypertension, moderate physical activity can lower your blood pressure.

4. **REDUCE YOUR SALT INTAKE** to no more than about 1 teaspoon of table salt (or 2.4 grams of sodium) per day. Many people are salt-sensitive when it comes to their blood pressure. Reducing the amount of salt you consume may gradually reduce both your blood pressure and, for those on drugs, the amount of blood pressure–lowering medication you need to take. Even if you cannot get down to 1 teaspoon, lowering your salt intake by any amount can still make a difference. It's not enough simply to use less salt from the salt shaker at the dinner table: 75 percent of the salt we ingest comes from processed food. Check the sodium content on the nutrition labels of everything you buy at the grocery store, and ask about salt content when ordering in restaurants.

5. **QUIT SMOKING.** Blood pressure goes up when you smoke. Smoking may also prevent you from getting the full benefit of blood pressure–lowering medications.

Lowering Blood Pressure with Medication

If your blood pressure is higher than the "pre-hypertension" range—that is, if it is classified as either Stage 1 or 2 hypertension—your doctor will likely recommend not only these lifestyle changes but will also prescribe medication treatment.

Some of the medications used to treat other heart-related problems may also be prescribed just for high blood pressure. These drugs include beta-blockers, calcium channel–blockers, and angiotensin-converting enzyme (ACE) inhibitors and are described in more detail later in this chapter. But several recent studies have demonstrated that thiazide diuretics, inexpensive medications that have been around for a long time, are as good as newer and more expensive drugs for lowering blood pressure. Thiazide diuretics, such as hydrochlorothiazide (sometimes called HCTZ), can cause you to urinate more. Their effect on blood pressure occurs after being on the drug for a short time. A recent clinical study of more than 30,000 people with hypertension showed that thiazide diuretics were as effective (and less expensive) for protecting against heart problems, stroke, and narrowing of the arteries than ACE inhibitors or calcium channel-blockers. These findings received a lot of media attention, but another new study showed that ACE inhibitors work better than diuretics at protecting against future heart problems and death. So there remains some controversy about the best approach.

New studies comparing antihypertension medications are coming out all the time. In a recent clinical study involving people with long-standing hypertension, a relatively new medication called an *angiotensin receptor-blocker* (ARB) lowered blood pressure just as well as beta-blockers. Furthermore, ARBs prevented even more heart attacks, strokes, and deaths than the beta-blockers over the long term. These benefits were especially strong for people with diabetes.

Conflicting studies can be confusing for physicians and their patients. Even as doctors debate the best approach, you should know that there remains strong agreement that the control of blood pressure is what is most important.

For now, the Joint National Committee on High Blood Pressure recommends that patients who need medication for high blood pressure first be considered for a thiazide diuretic and then an ACE inhibitor, ARB, beta-blocker, or calcium channel–blocker, or a combination of these drugs. The committee also recommends that patients with Stage 2 hypertension be started on two medications from the beginning, preferably a thiazide diuretic in combination with another class of blood pressure–lowering medication.

To make this clear, here's what you really need to know:

- There are proven medications for lowering your blood pressure, and precisely which medication is right for you is something you need to explore with your doctor.

- If you're taking medication but it fails to reduce your blood pressure enough to reach your target levels, talk to your doctor. Your doctor should increase the dose or add another medication. Sometimes, taking more than one type of medication is the only way to bring your blood pressure down to target range. If your blood pressure is still too high despite taking medication, don't increase the dose without talking to your doctor.

- If you are taking more than one prescription, over-the-counter, or alternative medicine at a time, be sure to ask your doctor or pharmacist about potential negative interactions. You can turn to pages 181–186 for a summary of common drug interactions. It's your responsibility to make sure your doctors are aware of all the medicines you take. You should have a list that you bring to each visit.

Blood Pressure Medication Side Effects

Like all medications, those used to treat high blood pressure have potential side effects. Most of these side effects are specific to the particular family of medication you may be taking. One uncommon side effect that all of these medications can cause is "hypotension," having a blood pressure that is too low. Older adults may be more prone to periods of hypotension, especially after rising quickly or after eating a meal. Symptoms typically involve feeling dizzy or light-headed for a brief period of time. These symptoms can be reduced by starting the medication at a very low dose and gradually increasing it until it reaches an effective level. You should talk with your doctor if you feel dizzy or light-headed.

Common Side Effects of Blood Pressure–Lowering Medications	
Medication	**Common Side Effects**
thiazide diuretics	increased frequency of urination; for this reason, many people find it more convenient to take their pill in the morning so that they are not bothered by this side effect at night
ACE inhibitors	dry cough (see section on ACE inhibitors), elevated potassium
ARBs	dry cough, elevated potassium
calcium channel–blockers	depends on the type of calcium channel–blocker; possibilities include: headache, ankle swelling
beta-blockers	slow heart rate, fatigue (see section on beta-blockers)

Adapted from the sixth report of the Joint National Committee on Prevention, Detection, Evaluation, and Treatment of High Blood Pressure, National Institutes of Health, National Heart, Lung, and Blood Institute, 1997.

Making Blood Pressure Medications Work for You

Ironically, the most common reason high blood pressure medications don't work is that patients don't take them. In a sense, this isn't surprising. High blood pressure has few symptoms; it's easy for people to forget to take their medication. But make no mistake: high blood pressure is dangerous; not taking your medication is inviting trouble. If you're taking your medication as prescribed and your blood pressure still hasn't changed appreciably, or if the side effects of the medication make you want to stop taking it, you should talk to your doctor about switching to a different medication.

That raises an important question: Can you ever stop taking hypertension medication? Yes, it's entirely possible. If your blood pressure has been under control for at least one year, your doctor may decide it is possible to reduce the dose you're taking—in time, perhaps, to zero. But this should be done slowly and gradually. This "step-down" therapy is most successful in people who have made and maintained the lifestyle changes that can bring high blood pressure under control. When you reach this point you may want to talk to your doctor about working together to see if you can reduce or eliminate your medications. If you're able to work with your doctor to stop your medications, you will still need to monitor your blood pressure carefully, because it can rise again, even months or years later—especially if you abandon those lifestyle changes.

Frequently Asked Questions

Q: WHICH IS MORE IMPORTANT—SYSTOLIC OR DIASTOLIC BLOOD PRESSURE?

It's important to control both systolic and diastolic blood pressure. For many years doctors focused mostly on the diastolic blood pressure (the "bottom" number). However, studies have found that in people over age fifty, a high systolic blood pressure is more closely related to heart disease, stroke, kidney disease, and death. People know now that it is best to pay attention to both.

Q: WHAT IF I HAVE TROUBLE ONLY WITH MY SYSTOLIC BLOOD PRESSURE?

Many people have normal diastolic pressure but hard-to-control systolic pressure. This is especially common among older adults.

Thiazide diuretics (for example, hydrochlorothiazide or HCTZ) and calcium channel–blockers have been shown to work especially well in these situations. But other medications can also work for people who have high systolic blood pressure, and so it is generally recommended that the same approach to lowering blood pressure overall be used for people with hard-to-control systolic pressure.

Q: CAN A BLOOD PRESSURE BE TOO LOW?
While blood pressure that's too high is dangerous, low blood pressure also can cause symptoms, though typically not dangerous ones. If your blood pressure is too low, you may feel dizzy, tired, or weak. This usually does not happen until the systolic blood pressure goes below 100 mmHg. If you have these symptoms, you should definitely talk with your doctor about them. Many people have even lower blood pressure without any symptoms.

Q: WHAT ABOUT CALCIUM, POTASSIUM, OR MAGNESIUM SUPPLEMENTS?
No medical consensus has emerged yet to support taking any of these supplements to lower blood pressure. The few studies that favor taking supplements are not scientifically strong. What we do know is that not having enough of these nutrients in your regular diet may increase your blood pressure. So, to optimize your overall health as well as your blood pressure level, you should ensure you are incorporating adequate amounts of these nutrients into a healthy balanced diet. (See the DASH Diet on pages 26–30.)

Q: WHAT ABOUT EPHEDRA?
Ephedra, the herbal compound also known as "ma huang," is an ingredient in some weight-loss supplements. It is closely related to ephedrine and pseudoephedrine, medications contained in some decongestants, bronchodilators, and stimulants. Concerns have been raised about the potential for these drugs to cause hypertension, heart attack, and stroke. The Food and Drug Administration (FDA) banned dietary supplements that contain ephedra. However, the ban excludes the use of the herb in traditional Asian med-

icine. The FDA ruling considers herbal medicine preparations beyond the scope of its authority. As a result, ephedra will not disappear. Therefore, if you already have high blood pressure, diabetes, or heart disease, you should not take medications containing ephedra. If you regularly use herbal medicines or tea, you should check to see if they contain ephedra.

Q: WHAT ABOUT CAFFEINE?

Caffeine may increase your blood pressure right after you drink it, which is why you should avoid caffeine before having your blood pressure measured. But drinking a lot of caffeine has not been shown to raise your blood pressure over the long term.

Q: IS HIGH BLOOD PRESSURE HARDER TO CONTROL IN AFRICAN-AMERICANS?

For reasons that we do not yet fully understand, hypertension develops earlier in African-Americans, and their average blood pressure tends to be higher. African-Americans have higher rates of Stage 2 hypertension and therefore are more prone to complications. The good news is that the combination of lifestyle changes and medication works just as well to reduce blood pressure for African-Americans as for everybody else. In fact, studies show that the DASH Diet (see pages 26–30) is even more effective in African-Americans than in others. The diet alone works as well to treat Stage 1 hypertension as using a medication. Some studies suggest that certain medications, such as ACE inhibitors and ARBs, are not as effective in African-Americans as they are in others. However, these studies are considered controversial and you should know that current expert consensus is that all blood pressure–lowering medications work for African-Americans. As with all patients, what is important is to be persistent in treating high blood pressure and to monitor the effects of therapy.

Q: DOES STRESS CAUSE HIGH BLOOD PRESSURE?

Blood pressure tends to go up when we are stressed and then go down when we are relaxed. Being stressed on a frequent or chronic basis may have something to do with developing hypertension, but the data are not definitive. Some researchers have theorized that including stress-management techniques or quiet periods of meditation in your daily or weekly routine may help to lower blood pressure, along with other heart problems. If stress is a problem for you, stress-management techniques may help you feel better and will likely pose no harm, so this approach may be worth a try. However, the jury is still out on whether or not they can substitute for the other lifestyle and medication treatments in managing your blood pressure.

Q: WHAT IS "WHITE COAT HYPERTENSION"?

If your blood pressure is high every time it is measured in your doctor's office or similar medical setting, but low whenever it is measured anywhere else, you may have what is called "white coat hypertension." Some people become anxious in a doctor's office and their blood pressure rises. While some experts question the concept of white coat hypertension, the prevailing belief is that the stress that causes it is real—and that people who experience it experience it at other stressful times as well. Therefore, many experts currently recommend that people with white coat hypertension be treated like other people with high blood pressure.

Q: WHAT IS "AMBULATORY BLOOD PRESSURE MONITORING"?

Ambulatory blood pressure monitoring, sometimes called ABPM for short, is a test in which a patient wears a blood pressure–measuring device continuously for a twenty-four-hour period to record blood pressure throughout the day and night. This test is often used to evaluate white coat hypertension, but it can also be used to investigate hypertension that does not seem to respond to medication, blood pressure that drops too low during medication treatment, and blood pressure that appears to fluctuate with unusual patterns.

Q: HOW OFTEN SHOULD I MONITOR MY BLOOD PRESSURE?

When you are having your medications changed, you should have your blood pressure monitored every few weeks. Once your blood pressure has stabilized, you can measure it less frequently, but many people find that frequent measurements help them to maintain their motivation. The only caveat is that blood pressure can vary from day to day.

★★ The DASH Diet

Clinical studies have proven that the Dietary Approaches to Stop Hypertension (DASH) Diet lowers blood pressure. The DASH Diet is rich in fruits, vegetables, and low-fat dairy foods. Therefore, it's low in total and saturated fat as well as cholesterol, and high in fiber, potassium, calcium, magnesium, and protein.

Below is a sample 2,000-calorie-per-day DASH Diet eating plan. It can be varied depending upon your caloric intake needs.

The DASH Diet				
Food Group	Daily Serving	Serving Sizes	Examples and Notes	Significance of Each Group Food to the DASH Diet
Grains and grain products	7–8	1 slice bread, ½ cup dry cereal; ½ cup cooked rice, pasta, or cereal	whole-wheat bread, English muffin, pita bread, bagel, cereals, grits, oatmeal	major sources of energy and fiber
Vegetables	4–5	1 cup raw leafy vegetable; ½ cup cooked vegetable; 6 oz. vegetable juice	tomatoes, potatoes, carrots, peas, squash, broccoli, turnip greens, collards, kale, spinach, artichokes, beans, sweet potatoes	rich sources of potassium, magnesium, and fiber
Fruits	4–5	6 oz. fruit juice; 1 medium fruit; ¼ cup dried fruit; ¼ cup fresh,	apricots, bananas, dates, grapes, oranges, orange juice, grapefruit,	important sources of potassium, magnesium,

Food Group	Daily Serving	Serving Sizes	Examples and Notes	Significance of Each Group Food to the DASH Diet
Fruits (*continued*)		frozen, or canned fruit	grapefruit juice, mangoes, melons, peaches, pineapples, prunes, raisins, strawberries, tangerines	and fiber
Low-fat or nonfat dairy foods	2–3	8 oz. milk; 1 cup yogurt; 1.5 oz. cheese	skim or 1% milk, skim or low-fat buttermilk, nonfat or low-fat yogurt, part-skim mozzarella cheese, nonfat cheese	major sources of calcium and protein
Meats, poultry, and fish	2 or less	3 oz. cooked meats, poultry, or fish	select only lean; trim away visible fats; broil, roast, or boil (instead of frying); remove skin from poultry	rich sources of protein and magnesium
Nuts, seeds, and legumes	4–5 per week	1.5 oz. or ⅓ cup nuts; ½ oz. or 2 Tbsp. seeds; ½ cup cooked legumes	almonds, filberts, mixed nuts, peanuts, walnuts, sunflower seeds, kidney beans, lentils	rich sources of energy, magnesium, potassium, protein, and fiber

Adapted from the sixth report of the Joint National Committee on Prevention, Detection, Evaluation, and Treatment of High Blood Pressure, National Institutes of Health, National Heart, Lung, and Blood Institute, 1997.

Sample Menu Based on a 2,000 Calories/Day Diet

Food	Amount	Servings Provided
BREAKFAST		
orange juice	6 oz.	1 fruit
low-fat (1%) milk	8 oz. (1 cup)	1 dairy
corn flakes (with 1 tsp. sugar)	1 cup	2 grains
banana	1 medium	1 fruit
whole-wheat bread (with 1 Tbsp. jelly)	1 slice	1 grain
soft margarine	1 tsp.	1 fat
LUNCH		
chicken salad	¾ cup	1 poultry
pita bread	½, large	1 grain
raw vegetable medley: carrot and celery sticks	3–4 sticks ea.	1 vegetable
radishes	2	
loose-leaf lettuce	2 leaves	
part-skim mozzarella cheese	1½ slices	1 dairy
low-fat (1%) milk	8 oz. (1 cup)	1 dairy
fruit cocktail in light syrup	½ cup	1 fruit
DINNER		
herbed baked cod	3 oz.	1 fish
scallion rice	1 cup	2 grains
steamed broccoli	½ cup	1 vegetable
stewed tomatoes	½ cup	1 vegetable
spinach salad: raw spinach	½ cup	1 vegetable
cherry tomatoes	2	½ fat
cucumber	2 slices	1 grain
light Italian salad dressing	1 Tbsp.	1 fat
whole-wheat dinner roll	1 small	1 fruit
soft margarine	1 tsp.	
melon balls	½ cup	

Food	Amount	Servings Provided
SNACKS		
dried apricots	1 oz. (¼ cup)	1 fruit
mini-pretzels	1 oz. (¾ cup)	1 grain
mixed nuts	1.5 oz. (⅓ cup)	1 nut
diet ginger ale	12 oz.	0

Adapted from the sixth report of the Joint National Committee on Prevention, Detection, Evaluation, and Treatment of High Blood Pressure, National Institutes of Health, National Heart, Lung, and Blood Institute, 1997.

Total Number of Servings in a 2,000 Calories/Day Menu

FOOD GROUP	NUMBER OF SERVINGS
Grains	8
Vegetables	4
Fruits	5
Dairy Foods	3
Meats, Poultry, and Fish	2
Nuts, Seeds, and Legumes	1
Fats and Oils	2.5

Tips on Eating the DASH Way

1. Start small. Make gradual changes in your eating habits.
2. Center your meal around carbohydrates, such as pasta, rice, beans, or vegetables.
3. Treat meat as one part of the whole meal, instead of the focus.
4. Use fruits or low-fat, low-calorie foods such as sugar-free gelatin for desserts and snacks.

REMEMBER! If you use the DASH Diet to help prevent or control high blood pressure, make it part of a lifestyle that includes choosing foods

(continued)

lower in salt and sodium, keeping a healthy weight, being physically active, and, if you drink alcohol, doing so in moderation.

Adapted from the sixth report of the Joint National Committee on Prevention, Detection, Evaluation, and Treatment of High Blood Pressure, National Institutes of Health, National Heart, Lung, and Blood Institute, 1997.

You can find out more about this diet from the National Institutes of Health website at http://www.nhlbi.nih.gov/health/public/heart/hbp/dash/

Strategy #2:
★★★ Take Charge of Your Cholesterol

There are few things in modern medicine clearer than the link between cholesterol and heart disease. Over the last decade, research studies involving thousands of patients with heart disease have shown that lowering cholesterol decreases your risk of having a heart attack by as much as 40 percent.

Cholesterol is a substance your body actually needs. It's important in the production of certain hormones, including estrogen and testosterone, and it helps maintain the integrity of the walls of all the cells in your body. Cholesterol is produced in the liver from the foods we eat—mainly fats, but also proteins and carbohydrates. It can also come directly from foods containing cholesterol. But even though it is an essential substance, as many as 100 million Americans—nearly half of all adults—may have too much of it in their bloodstream. Even so, one-third of people with high cholesterol have no idea they have it. Of those who do know, only one-third are being treated for their high cholesterol, and fewer than half of people receiving treatment have been treated enough to bring their cholesterol levels into safe range.

Excess cholesterol collects on the insides of the artery walls in fatty streaks. It's one of the primary constituents of the plaques that cause arteries to narrow and "harden," making them vulnerable both to rupture and blockage. As we've seen, when this occurs in arteries supplying the heart, it can damage the heart. We normally think of this process as occurring in older adults, but in fact it begins at an early age. Autopsies of American soldiers killed in the Korean War first alerted doctors to the fact that even healthy young men already have some fatty streaks, or atherosclerotic plaque buildup in their blood vessels. We now know that many people have fatty streaks by age twenty—or even earlier.

As with high blood pressure, high cholesterol has no obvious symptoms; most of the people who have cholesterol levels that are too high don't even know it. The good news is that—again, like high blood pressure—high cholesterol can be diagnosed and treated. Yet as many as two-thirds of the people with high cholesterol go untreated.

Getting Your Cholesterol Tested

The only way to find out if your cholesterol levels are too high is to have a blood test called a "lipid panel." This test typically measures four things:

- **LDL (LOW-DENSITY LIPOPROTEIN) CHOLESTEROL** Cholesterol is composed of proteins and fats. LDL cholesterol has a low density, or low concentration, of protein but a high density of the fats that cause atherosclerosis. It's also known as "bad" cholesterol.

- **HDL (HIGH-DENSITY LIPOPROTEIN) CHOLESTEROL** HDL cholesterol has a high density of protein and relatively little fat. It collects excess fat in your bloodstream and carries it to the liver for disposal. It's a sort of fat scavenger. That's why it's known as "good" cholesterol. If your HDL is low, those excess fats build up instead of being removed.

- **TOTAL CHOLESTEROL** This is a total measure of the cholesterol in your blood and includes LDL and HDL cholesterol as well as some other cholesterol components.

- **TRIGLYCERIDES** These are another form of fat the body makes from sugar, alcohol, or extra calories.

All four of these measurements provide useful information, but by far the most important for people with heart disease is LDL cholesterol, because that's the one most closely linked to atherosclerosis and the one that can be most easily treated.

What Do the Guidelines Say?

Based on strong evidence from many clinical studies, heart experts have developed targets for your cholesterol levels (usually reported in milligrams per deciliter, or mg/dL):

- LDL cholesterol should be under 100 mg/dL for patients with heart disease (or 70 mg/dL for very high risk patients)
- HDL cholesterol should be 40 mg/dL or higher
- Total cholesterol should be below 200 mg/dL
- Triglycerides should be below 150 mg/dL

Recent clinical trials have caused the National Cholesterol Education Program, the authoritative group of experts that is convened by the National Heart, Lung, and Blood Institute of the National Institutes of Health, to revise their recommendation for the target level of LDL cholesterol. The goal for people with heart disease remains less than 100 mg/dL, but now they also endorse a target of less than 70 mg/dL for high-risk patients, which includes patients with established heart disease. The new target is called an option, or a "reasonable clinical strategy."

The revised recommendations say that an LDL of less than 70 mg/dL is a reasonable clinical strategy on the basis of available clinical evidence, and an LDL of less than 100 mg/dL remains the strong recommendation. The guidelines indicate that the lower target is particularly favored for patients with established heart disease *and* either (1) other major risk factors (such as diabetes); or (2) severe and poorly controlled risk factors (including continued smoking); or (3) high triglycerides (200 mg/dL or greater) and non-HDL cholesterol of 130 mg/dL or greater with an HDL of 40 mg/dL or lower; or (4) hospitalization for a heart attack.

The reason that they are not stronger in recommending the level of less than 70 mg/dL is that several studies are in progress to evaluate reducing the LDL to very low levels. The principal reason for the recommendation change is the Pravastatin or Atorvastatin Evaluation and Infection Therapy (PROVE-IT) trial, which found that patients benefit from lowering cholesterol levels below the old target. Over 4,000 patients who were hospitalized with heart disease were randomized to a high dose (80 mg) of atorvastatin or a standard dose (40 mg) of pravastatin. With the high dose of atorvastatin, the LDL was lowered to around 62 mg/dL, whereas the standard dose of pravastatin lowered the LDL to about 95 mg/dL. The more aggressive approach was associated with a 16 percent reduction over two years in the risk of cardiovascular events. The advantage of the more aggressive strategy is what led to this change in the recommendation.

Lowering Cholesterol with Lifestyle Changes

If your LDL cholesterol is between 100 and 130, the current guidelines say that you should aim to lower it through lifestyle changes—that is, through diet, exercise, and weight management—before moving to medications. As with blood pressure control, the first step has to do with lifestyle.

DIET   Scientists believe that the amount of fat you eat is directly related to how high your LDL cholesterol level is. But there are many different kinds of fats. Understanding the differences between types of fats is so important to preventing and controlling heart disease that this book provides a separate discussion of the issue in a special section called Managing Your Diet (see pages 109–124). In general, however, the American Heart Association (AHA) guidelines suggest that you limit your overall fat intake to less than 30 percent of your total daily calories. Of that total 30 percent, saturated fats should represent less than 7 percent. Cutting fat works: researchers have shown that a low-fat diet can lower

LDL cholesterol levels by 7 to 9 percent in people with high cholesterol.

The AHA experts also recommend increasing your consumption of vegetables that contain LDL cholesterol–lowering monounsaturated fatty acids and fiber. Fatty acids are labeled based on their chemical structure. Monounsaturated fatty acids are a major nutrient in the food supply of the Mediterranean countries. Olive oil and canola oil are examples of high monounsaturated fatty acid foods. Current evidence also suggests that eating more foods that contain omega-3 fatty acids, found in many kinds of fish, also can protect you from heart problems. Salmon is an example of a high omega-3 fatty acid food.

EXERCISE   Physical activity increases HDL cholesterol and lowers LDL cholesterol. Indeed, one recent study showed that increased exercise alone can significantly improve your cholesterol profile. The recommended goal for exercise is moderately intense physical activity (the equivalent of briskly walking at three to four miles per hour for most healthy adults) for thirty minutes per day, at least five times per week. Of course, how much you can exercise depends on your overall health, so talk to your doctor about a program that's best for you.

WEIGHT MANAGEMENT   If you are overweight—and many Americans are—losing even a few pounds will lower your LDL cholesterol. This is true regardless of what you eat, but a calorie-controlled diet that is low in saturated fats and cholesterol is best; it will help all other efforts to lower your LDL cholesterol and help keep it low over time.

Lowering Cholesterol with Medication

Sometimes lifestyle changes alone will not bring your cholesterol to healthy levels and medication is required. A decade or so ago, the medications available for reducing cholesterol had only limited effectiveness and often produced unpleasant side effects.

STATINS   More recently, however, scientists have developed and successfully tested a class of drugs called *statins*, which both slow the production of cholesterol and increase the liver's ability to remove LDL cholesterol already in your bloodstream. They also reduce your triglyceride levels and can often moderately increase your HDL cholesterol levels. They are extremely effective, are very safe, and people taking them rarely experience side effects at recommended dosages.

A number of large clinical trials have shown that when people with heart disease take statins, their cholesterol levels not only go down, but their risk for other heart problems or stroke drops sharply as well. For example, statins can lower your risk of heart attack by up to 40 percent, lower your chance of needing heart surgery by up to 40 percent, lower your risk of stroke by at least 20 percent (and up to 55 percent), and lower your risk of death by up to 30 percent. And that's not all. Another recent clinical study involving more than 20,000 people showed that statins can cut the risk of heart attack and stroke by a third in people with a high risk for heart problems *even if they had low or normal cholesterol levels to begin with*.

All of this research suggests that statins may have a protective effect on the heart in addition to lowering cholesterol. What's more, there is evidence that statins may benefit your brain as well as your heart: statins decrease your risk of stroke, of course, but research now suggests that they may also help prevent Alzheimer's disease.

Consequently, even though the expert guidelines currently recommend drug therapy only after lifestyle modification has failed, statins have proven so effective that many doctors have begun to encourage their use right from the start, in addition to lifestyle management.

There are several statin drugs on the market today. Although *simvastatin* and *pravastatin* have been tested the most and other statins have been studied less thoroughly, all appear to have the same benefits for a given reduction in LDL. Still, some of their properties differ:

Special Properties of Certain Statins

simvastatin; pravastatin; atorvastatin	most studied in clinical trials
atorvastatin; rosuvastatin	most effective at lowering LDL cholesterol levels
atorvastatin; fluvastatin	least affected by kidney problems
pravastatin; fluvastatin	least likely to interact with other medications
fluvastatin; atorvastatin; lovastatin	most cost-effective for the amount by which they lower LDL cholesterol levels

Commonly Used Statins and Their Brand Names

Generic Name	Brand Name	Standard Dose
atorvastatin	Lipitor	10–80 mg/day*
fluvastatin	Lescol	20–80 mg/day*
lovastatin	Mevacor	20–80 mg/day*
pravastatin	Pravachol	40–80 mg/day*
rosuvastatin	Crestor	5–40 mg/day†
simvastatin	Zocor	5–80 mg/day*

* available up to 80 mg
† available up to 40 mg

As with any prescription, you should talk to your doctor about other drugs you are taking before beginning statin treatment. Some people experience negative reactions when they combine statins with other medications, though most of these reactions are rare. If you have concerns, you should talk with your doctor.

SIDE EFFECTS OF STATINS   Most people taking statins experience no side effects at all. Of those who do, the most common are mild stomach upset, gas, nausea, diarrhea, constipation, or muscle weakness. More serious reactions, which can include liver damage or muscle breakdown, are possible but rare. However, the American Heart Association advises that patients have a creatine kinase (or CK) blood test (a test of muscle damage) before starting statins and any time signs of muscle damage appear, suggested by dark urine or severe muscle pain, tenderness, or weakness (though it is possible to have statin-related muscle problems even with a normal CK level).

Two other tests that measure blood levels of two specific liver markers, called AST (short for: aspartate aminotransferase) and ALT (short for: alanine aminotransferase), should be done three months after beginning statin drugs and then at least once a year afterward, or any time a patient shows signs of possible liver disease (excessive fatigue, nausea, and vomiting).

Although these tests for kidney and liver function are recommended for everybody taking a statin, you should know that the overall risk of developing signs of kidney or liver problems while taking a statin is less than 1 percent (that's less than one in one hundred).

Drinking grapefruit juice can increase the effect of some statins, including simvastatin, atorvastatin, and lovastatin (but not pravastatin). Grapefruit seems to inhibit the enzymes that break down some of the statins. This makes it difficult to be sure how much medication you are getting with each dose. Nevertheless, for people taking their statin at night, a small glass of grapefruit juice in the morning is unlikely to cause a problem.

An issue that is currently under investigation is the impact of statins on behavior and memory. Some researchers are looking into this issue. At this time there is not yet enough evidence to support this concern.

Other Cholesterol Drugs

Statins are the first choice for treating high cholesterol because of the overwhelming evidence supporting their effectiveness. If you cannot take statins, other medications can help you bring your cholesterol under control. In fact, because of their special properties, some of these alternatives are occasionally prescribed with statins.

BILE ACID RESINS are not quite as powerful as statins at lowering LDL cholesterol or raising HDL cholesterol, but they can decrease cholesterol levels. Bile acid resins (e.g., cholestyramine [brand names: Cholybar, LoCholest, LoCholest Light, Prevalite, Questran, Questran Light], colestipol [brand name: Colestid], and colesevelam [brand name: Welchol]) are very safe and can be added to statins to help lower LDL cholesterol. These medications never became very popular—probably because they can cause constipation, bloating, nausea, or gas and need to be taken with a lot of fluid.

NICOTINIC ACID, commonly known as niacin or vitamin B_3, is not as effective at lowering LDL cholesterol as statins, but is better at raising HDL cholesterol and may be better at lowering triglycerides. It is inexpensive and does not require a prescription, but a common side effect is facial flushing or hot flashes that some people find intolerable. The prescription long-acting forms tend to be better tolerated. As an interesting note, niacin deficiency used to cause a disease called pellagra, which was characterized by problems with the skin, digestive system, and nervous system. With dietary improvements, this disease is no longer a problem in the United States.

FIBRATES (e.g., gemfibrozil [brand name: Lopid], fenofibrate [brand name: Tricor], and clofibrate [brand name: Atromid]) are not as effective at lowering LDL cholesterol as statins, but because they are slightly better than statins at raising HDL cholesterol and much better for lowering triglycerides, the two are sometimes combined. Side effects of fibrates, though uncommon, include nausea, diarrhea, stomach upset, heartburn, and gas. Also, in rare instances, fibrates may cause kidney or muscle problems in people taking statins and may increase the risk of bleeding in people taking blood thinners unless the dose is adjusted.

The interesting thing about fibrates is that studies have found that their modest ability to increase HDL may translate into substantial benefits for patients. In a study of more than 2,500 veterans, gemfibrozil increased HDL levels by 6 percent, reduced total cholesterol by 4 percent, and reduced triglycerides by 31 percent. Over the five years of the study, gemfibrozil was associated with a 22 percent reduction in the risk of heart attacks and death.

SELECTIVE CHOLESTEROL ABSORPTION INHIBITOR (e.g., ezetimibe [brand name: Zetia]) is a medicine that works in the intestine. It is generally well tolerated and can be helpful for patients who cannot take statins. Also, many doctors are using it in combination with statin drugs. A recent study suggests that the coadministration of ezetimibe and statin therapy is more effective in reducing LDL cholesterol than statin therapy alone. There is much less information about the long-term effects of this medication. Whether this strategy is better than increasing the dose of the statin is not known. Ezetimibe should not be taken by patients also taking bile acid resins because the bile acid resins may bind to it and make it ineffective.

Frequently Asked Questions

Q: WHAT IF MY TOTAL CHOLESTEROL IS AT TARGET BUT MY LDL IS STILL ABOVE TARGET?

It's a common misunderstanding among patients that total cholesterol is more important than LDL and HDL cholesterol. In fact, it's just the opposite. Your LDL needs to be below 100 (or 70) for your cholesterol levels to be at target. If your total cholesterol is low despite the fact that your LDL cholesterol is high, it may mean that your HDL cholesterol is too low.

Q: MY LDL CHOLESTEROL IS GOING DOWN BUT MY HDL CHOLESTEROL WILL NOT GO UP. WHAT CAN I DO?

If you have heart disease, it is particularly important that your HDL cholesterol be as high as possible—at least 40 mg/dL. A lower HDL cholesterol level can be a result of your being overweight, physically inactive, or a smoker. Addressing these issues is the first step to raising your HDL. Beyond this, you and your doctor may decide to use medication (such as fibrates or niacin) to help raise your HDL. In the end, your HDL target may still be hard to reach. Researchers are currently working on products that may specifically target the HDL cholesterol level.

Q: CAN EATING MORE FIBER, NUTS, SOY, OR GARLIC LOWER MY CHOLESTEROL?

There is not enough evidence to support using any of these foods as first-line approaches to lowering cholesterol. For more information about the effect of certain types of foods on cholesterol, turn to the Managing Your Diet section on pages 109–124.

Q: DOES IT MATTER WHEN I TAKE STATINS?

Doctors generally recommend that patients take statins in a single dose at dinner or at bedtime. By taking the medication at this time you take advantage of the fact that the body manufactures more cholesterol at night than during the day.

Q: HOW LONG DOES IT TAKE TO SEE THE EFFECTS OF STATINS?

Patients usually see the results of statins fairly soon after starting the medication—and the maximum effect is usually seen by four to six weeks. Doctors usually recheck cholesterol levels about six to eight weeks after initiating therapy.

Strategy #3:
★★★ Take Charge of Your Fitness

Few things in life make an otherwise healthy person feel more fragile than a diagnosis of heart disease. Even without having had a heart attack, the sober announcement by your family doctor that you have heart disease is usually a deeply unnerving event. Suddenly, you feel quite vulnerable. Instinct may tell you the best and safest thing to do is go home, lie down, and have a good long rest. Let the heart repair itself.

For decades, doctors had the same instinct. They often kept patients at rest in the hospital or at home for weeks. But researchers have discovered this instinct was wrong: exercise is *good* for the heart. It may be most important for people who have heart disease. Studies show that, in people with heart disease, exercise-based rehabilitation strengthens the heart and helps it to work more efficiently. In fact, for people with heart disease, doing exercise as part of a rehabilitation program is associated with a 25 percent lower risk of having a fatal heart attack or stroke.

Why? Because exercise doesn't just strengthen the heart muscle itself; it improves the health of your arteries and the rest of your cardiovascular system, too. In the process it reduces the likelihood that clots will form that might trigger a heart attack. Exercise lowers blood pressure and increases HDL (good) cholesterol levels, keeps blood sugar under control, and increases overall endurance. It is true that people who exercise sometimes have heart problems, but this occurs far less frequently than it does in people who don't exercise.

What's more, research demonstrates that participating in an exercise program even *after* a heart attack may lower your chances of dying from a heart problem by 20 to 30 percent. A study of 21,000 people has shown that men who exercised enough to work up a sweat at least once a week were 20 percent less likely to have a stroke. A study of women found that walking briskly at least three hours a week cut their risk of heart disease by 30 to 40 percent. Indeed, exercise even fights the depression that often follows a heart disease diagnosis or a heart attack. After all, it's hard to keep thinking of yourself as fragile when you're working up a sweat.

Does that mean the first thing you should do after your diagnosis is start vigorous exercise? Of course not. But guided by your doctor and an exercise professional, exercise is not only safe, it's critical to your long-term health. With a little imagination, it can even be fun—a lot more fun than another heart attack.

What the Guidelines Say

Health organizations like the Centers for Disease Control and Prevention and the National Institutes of Health now recommend that adults exercise at least 30 minutes every day. The Institute of Medicine, an authoritative group of medical experts, recently went even further: it recommends that all adults engage in at least 60 minutes of moderately intense physical activity most days of the week in order to maintain ideal body weight and gain all the other benefits that come with being active.

For those who can't meet these goals, however, the advice of all the experts is simple: "Some exercise is better than none, and more is better than some." These recommendations are not specifically for patients with heart disease, and they indicate a growing enthusiasm for encouraging physical activity.

The American Heart Association/American College of Cardiology guidelines recommend that people with heart disease do *at least* 30 minutes of aerobic exercise daily, or at a minimum three to four times a week. Aerobic (which means "oxygen demanding") exercise works large muscle groups in your body continuously over a period of time at a level vigorous enough to raise your heart rate. How you achieve this goal is up to you, with the guidance of your doctor. What's important is that you find a form of exercise, or combination of exercises, that you will want to keep up. Sure, joining a gym and working out on a treadmill, stair climber, or any of the many other aerobic exercise machines currently available will work. But so will dancing, bicycling, even walking, so long as you do it briskly and often enough.

And that's not all. The guidelines also recommend that in addition to working out, you modify your lifestyle in a way that makes your daily routine more active. For some heart disease patients this means skipping the coffee break and taking a walking break instead. Or taking the stairs instead of the elevator. Or being more actively involved in gardening. How you do it is up to you; what matters is that you do it.

Why Exercise Matters

The human body, and the heart that keeps it alive, were made for work. From the Stone Age until roughly fifty years ago, hard physical work was the norm for most people, as it still is today in many parts of the world where, in fact, heart disease is much less common. But during the twentieth century, as industrial societies became more technologically advanced, our lives became more sedentary. We went from hand scythes to push mowers, and from push mowers to power mowers, from power mowers to riding mowers, to pick just one example.

As we become more sedentary, we become more disease- and injury-prone. Muscles weaken. Weight piles on. Joints stiffen. Bone density decreases. The risk of disease—colon cancer, diabetes, anxiety, depression, and many more—increases sharply. At the top of the list is America's number-one killer, heart disease, and related conditions like high blood pressure and stroke. In short, our comfortable lives are killing us.

Many people don't exercise regularly. More than half of all Americans don't. Many don't exercise at all. We find lots of reasons not to exert ourselves. We don't have the time. Or the money. Or the equipment. But mostly, we don't have the will. In a society busily inventing new conveniences, it's increasingly easy to avoid physical work. We don't even have to leave the couch to change channels on our televisions. Our bodies may be designed for hard work, but, like pieces of equipment, if left idle too long they fall into disrepair.

Fortunately, it's almost never too late to start working your heart. Stated simply: the more exercise you get—even if it's only walking regularly—the lower your chance of having heart problems and the better your chance of beating them if you do. And if you have been exercising, then the goal is to get you back to your high level of activity—or more.

How Can I Put My Heart to Work?

Start, as always, with a talk with your doctor. Heart problems differ from individual to individual, and no one knows your heart's needs—your baseline condition and improvement targets—better than your doctor. You need to be safe as you start this program.

Any aerobic activity—that is, any form of exercise that raises your heart rate—will make your heart stronger in time. The more often you do it, the more fit your heart and blood vessels will be. The secret is to keep doing it. Most people, with or without heart disease, who start an exercise program don't keep at it. As many as half of all people who begin an exercise program have given it up within six months. When you have heart disease, you don't have that luxury. This isn't about losing weight or looking good; this is about staying alive.

How do you ensure you'll still be going strong—in fact, stronger—after six months? Simple, really: choose an exercise activity you really like, do well or can learn easily, and feel safe doing. Better yet, choose several. Make sure they can fit into your schedule and are affordable. Then make them part of your life. Give exercise priority and acknowledge its critical role in your recovery.

Some people like nothing better than to step onto a treadmill, get up to their target pace, and just go. Other people find treadmills tedious, every minute drudgery. If that's the case for you, give yourself something else to think about as you work your muscles and your heart. Listen to music. Watch a video. If that doesn't help, switch to another activity. Hate gyms and exercise machines? Fine. Go dancing. Or swimming. Or cycling.

The point is that it simply doesn't matter what you do to increase your aerobic activity; what matters is that you do it—a lot—and that you don't give it up. Choosing an activity you enjoy helps a lot. So does having an exercise partner. For one thing, it's nice to have company. For another, the days your partner doesn't feel like exercising will probably not be the same days you don't feel like it. On those days, you can each encourage the other. Nothing is quite like peer pressure to keep you on your toes. Researchers have found other techniques that can help you stick to the task as well.

For example, starting out with supervision helps you stay with the program over the long term. Images of your exercise goals will also help keep you on track. And committing, reminding and rewarding yourself, and focusing on what you are accomplishing turn out to be even more important than having fun or getting social support.

Don't underestimate the value of walking. Brisk walking is the most commonly prescribed form of aerobic activity for beginners. Almost anyone can do it, almost anywhere. Apart from a comfortable pair of shoes or sneakers, it requires no special equipment. It is, after all, something the human species is uniquely designed to do. You can do it alone, with a friend, or with a dog. It works: a recent study showed that brisk walking was associated with a marked reduction in the risk of heart disease. Note the word "brisk" here, however; ambling along casually does not do much to help your heart.

How Much Exercise Is Enough?

Good question. For most of us, the answer is, it's never "enough." Our lives are such today that we almost never get enough exercise to be as healthy and fit as we could be, or should be. Short of this ideal, however, here's what health experts agree will help fight heart disease:

HOW OFTEN?   At least three days a week of structured exercise, though every day is better. In addition, you should gradually increase the physical activity in your daily routine.

HOW LONG?   At least thirty minutes of aerobic activity every time you exercise. If you don't have thirty consecutive minutes, you can break it up into two fifteen-minute, or three ten-minute blocks.

HOW HARD?   Hard enough to get your heart rate up. Only then are you strengthening your cardiovascular system. To calculate your target heart rate for exercising, use the formula on page 47. Here's another gauge: you're working hard enough if you break into a sweat. A recent study found that exercise vigorous enough to cause you to sweat is related to reduced risk of stroke. How hard is too hard? Use the "talk test." If you can carry on a conversation while exercising, you're fine; if you can't, or if you're struggling to get out a sentence, chances are you need to slow down a bit (unless you are training to be an elite athlete).

KNOW WHEN TO STOP. If exercise begins to cause pain in your chest, arms, jaws, or stomach, sudden light-headedness or dizziness, cold sweats, nausea, vomiting, or weakness, call your doctor. If the symptoms persist after resting for five minutes, get medical help right away.

Beyond the Guideline Basics

The programs described in the preceding pages constitute the basic exercise regimen recommended by the American Heart Association/American College of Cardiology guidelines. Think of it as the bare minimum that will improve your condition. But the latest research suggests that a more comprehensive exercise program, involving longer aerobic conditioning as well as strength training, will produce greater benefits, not just for your heart but for your entire body. And that goes for people in every age group, including the elderly. Here's the basic structure:

- **WARM UP** (5 to 10 minutes). Do a low-level aerobic exercise (casual walking, slow treadmill, etc.) to increase cardiovascular activity and warm up muscles.

- **AEROBIC EXERCISE** (20 to 60 minutes). Walk briskly, jog, cycle, swim, do aerobic dancing, use a treadmill, stair climber, cross trainer, rower, or other exercise machine to elevate pulse to target heart rate. Begin gradually and increase the length of the workout over time to increase endurance (see page 170 for how to use an Exercise Log to chart your progress).

- **COOL DOWN** (5 to 10 minutes). Continue aerobic activity but at a gradually lower level of intensity. Many aerobic exercise machines build in a cool-down period automatically.

- **STRETCHING** (5 to 10 minutes). Gently stretch each major muscle group.

- **STRENGTH TRAINING** (15 to 30 minutes). Use weight-lifting machines, free weights, exercise bands (available from many doctors and clinics), or simply your own body for resistance (sit-ups, squats, push-ups, leg lifts) to do strength exercises for each major muscle group. Rotate muscle groups so that you do not work the same muscles on consecutive days.

- **FINAL STRETCHING** (5 to 10 minutes). Strength training can shorten muscles and tendons even as it strengthens them. Spend a few minutes gently stretching again at the end of your workout. Stretch slowly and hold each stretch for ten seconds. Don't bounce.

Remember to always consult your doctor before beginning an exercise program.

Know Your Target Heart Rate

When you exercise, your pulse, also called your heart rate, increases. To get the most from aerobic exercise, you should aim to increase your pulse to what's known as its "target rate," a figure between 60 and 80 percent of your heart's maximum rate per minute. What's your maximum heart rate per minute? Well, that varies, but a rough rule of thumb is to subtract your age from the number 220. If you're 60 years old, then, your maximum heart rate is 160 beats per minute and your target rate is in a zone between 96 and 128. But some medications, including so-called "beta-blockers," keep your heart rate low, so if you use these drugs, check with your doctor before estimating your target rate for exercise.

Frequently Asked Questions

Q: HOW DO I KNOW IF IT'S SAFE FOR ME TO EXERCISE?

You don't. But your doctor does. Before you begin any exercise program, consult your doctor. Your doctor may even recommend you take an exercise stress test to define your capacity to exercise. It isn't just safer to consult your doctor first, it's smart. It gives your doctor a chance to help you tailor the program to meet your specific needs, and to help you establish reasonable expectations. What's more, it gives you and your doctor an opportunity to establish fitness milestones against which to measure your progress. And measurable progress is a great motivator. If your doctor is not skilled at developing an exercise regimen, then he or she should refer you to someone who is.

Q: IS IT BETTER TO EXERCISE LONGER OR HARDER?
Longer is generally better than harder, but in the end both are important. If you spend too little time at it, you're not increasing your endurance. If you spend too little effort on it, you're not increasing your strength. And you need to do both. Here's an example: one study found that walking 3 to 4 miles an hour—that is, briskly enough to raise your heart rate—was as effective at lowering your risk of heart disease as vigorous exercise. But easy walking, the kind that does not increase your heart rate, had little effect. Their conclusion? How hard you walk—your pace—is as important as how long you walk.

Q: HOW DO I KNOW IF I'M EXERCISING TOO MUCH?
Do your joints or muscles hurt? Then you're probably exercising too hard, or too long. A certain amount of discomfort is normal; after all, these are muscles and body parts you haven't used much for a while. But if the discomfort is debilitating, or if it discourages you from keeping at it, then you're overdoing it. You may need to change the exercise you are doing. Also, getting fit again takes time, no matter what the magazines at the supermarket checkout stand claim. Be patient, be persistent, but be prudent, too; gradually increase how long and how hard you work out.

Q: WHAT ABOUT THOSE PEOPLE WHO HAVE HEART ATTACKS WHILE EXERCISING?
Yes, it's been known to happen. But rarely. And rarely to people who are exercising prudently. People who suffer heart problems

when doing aerobic exercises or lifting weights are often individuals who have been inactive for years and then throw themselves into strenuous workouts, instead of starting off slowly and building up gradually. The warning signs for heart trouble caused by overexercise are the same as those for heart trouble not triggered by exertion. But if you exercise prudently and regularly, the benefits far outstrip the risks.

Q: WHAT ABOUT WEIGHT LIFTING?

The most important form of exercise for your heart is aerobic. But weight lifting and other muscle-strengthening exercises (push-ups, sit-ups, squats, etc.) can also benefit your heart as well as your overall health. A recent study showed that men who weight-trained for at least thirty minutes per week had a 20 percent lower risk of heart disease. We also know that weight training can improve your endurance in aerobic workouts and reverse the atrophy, or weakening, of your muscles from years of inactivity—or simply advancing age. There is persuasive evidence that weight lifting increases bone density as well, in men and women alike. Most experts recommend that you do strength training at least twice a week, alternating with or complementing your aerobic workouts. But like everything else, this is best done in moderation.

HOW CAN I TELL IF THE EXERCISE IS WORKING?

It'll be obvious after a while. Your sense of vigor will grow and, as your physical health improves, your mental health will improve as well, partly because exercise releases "feel-good" chemicals in your brain. You'll also notice very real changes in the health of your heart. Your resting heart rate will decrease, and you'll return to your resting heart rate after exertion much more quickly. Your blood pressure will decrease, too. Initially, you may lose weight, which lessens the burden on your cardiovascular system. Don't be surprised, however, if after a while your weight increases a little even though your measurements are decreasing. Strong muscle weighs more (though it takes up less space) than fat.

WHAT IF I STOP EXERCISING?

You may, and for any number of reasons. Most people have lapses, so don't worry about it. Focus instead on how to get back into the groove again as soon as you can. If you stopped out of boredom, devise a new routine. Find an exercise partner. If you stopped for any reason, remember that you can't expect to go back and pick up where you left off. Muscles weaken quickly, even in an athlete, so start slowly and gradually build up to the level you reached before you stopped—and then keep going!

WHAT ABOUT WATCHING TELEVISION?

Television watching likely contributes to much of the sedentary behavior in our society. A study of 50,000 women found that their risk of obesity and diabetes could be predicted by the amount of time that they watched television. For each additional two hours a day of watching television, the participants had a 23 percent increase in the risk of obesity and a 14 percent increase in the risk of diabetes. The investigators estimated if Americans adopted a more active lifestyle with fewer than ten hours a week of television, then the incidence of obesity would drop 24 percent and diabetes would have a 34 percent reduction.

A PATIENT'S VIEW:
FINDING THE TIME

I am seventy-five years old and have been very active my whole life. I have three children and three grandchildren. I worked for many years as a secretary in an elementary school. Now I am involved with lots of volunteer work for different organizations. I'm definitely not the type of person who likes to sit still.

My health has generally been good. I have high blood pressure and high cholesterol but never thought too much about it. Last year I noticed that I was short of breath when I would walk up a hill. My children noticed that I was having trouble keeping up on a walk. I also noticed a discomfort in my throat. I thought that maybe I had a sore throat—but it only happened when I was exerting myself.

Finally I went to see my doctor who immediately sent me to a heart doctor. Before I knew it I was doing a treadmill test. After only about two minutes I started getting the sore throat again. I put my hands at the bottom of my throat and complained of the discomfort. The test was stopped and I remember the doctor telling me that I needed an angiogram. I was really shocked and told him that I had company coming that week and wanted to postpone the test. He told me that I needed the test that week—and that it could not wait. I listened carefully to every word and was petrified.

Although some others in my family had problems with their heart, I never considered it could happen to me. The day of the test my daughter was with me and we were both nervous. They found a large blockage and put in two stents to keep the artery open. I recovered quickly and then was told that I should go to cardiac rehabilitation sessions three times a week for twelve weeks. Wow. I remember wondering how I was ever going to fit that into my life.

At first I couldn't do much. I needed help with the treadmill. I was frustrated at the beginning. Day by day I gained strength. And it was not just the exercise. I took classes on nutrition. I met others who had gone through similar experiences.

How did I find the motivation to do it? I was scared. As much as I didn't want to give up the time, I wanted to survive. I made it my business to find the time. I want to live as long as I can and be as active as possible.

After the twelve weeks I joined a gym and now go three times a week. It is just a part of my routine. Also, I read everything I can about heart disease. I know that women can get heart disease, though many of us don't even realize it. You have to pay attention to your risk factors and your diet.

I also know the importance of my medications. I organize all of my pills each week. I don't like to take a lot of medications. I was never a person to take pills. I do it now. I question the need to take them on every doctor visit, but in the end I take what I am prescribed.

(continued)

> I definitely feel better than ever. Better than even before I knew that I had heart problems. I have more energy now. If you are in this situation you need to find the time.
> —Frances

Strategy #4:
★★★ Take Charge of Your Weight

Let's say I told you I'd created and patented a new pill that would lower your risk of heart disease, reduce your high blood pressure, cut your triglycerides, raise your level of HDL (good) cholesterol, lower your LDL (bad) cholesterol, reduce your risk of diabetes, and even lower your blood sugar levels to prevent or even reverse diabetes. You'd call it a miracle drug, for one thing. Then you'd call your pharmacist.

Well, there is no such miracle pill. That's the bad news. The good news is that I can prescribe something that will do all of these things, has no side effects, and is cheap as well. In fact, with this prescription, you'll probably end up actually saving money. Talk about miracles!

What's the miracle prescription? For people who are carrying extra pounds, it's weight reduction. That's right: the simple act of losing excess weight will do all these things.

So if you are carrying extra weight, you have a special opportunity to help yourself.

An Obesity Epidemic

Recent surveys estimate that almost two-thirds of all American adults are overweight or obese, and the numbers are increasing. A 2002 Harris Poll concluded that 80 percent of Americans over the age of twenty-five are overweight, up from less than 60 percent in 1983. And of those who are overweight, a third are very overweight (at least 20 percent overweight), a number that's doubled since 1983. The problem of excess weight and obesity is so widespread—

affecting men, women, and even children of all races and ethnic groups—and growing so quickly that the Surgeon General has termed it an epidemic and concluded that it's become a major health problem for the country.

We're not talking here about the discomfort of a belt that's a bit tight. The health consequences of overweight and obesity are profound: they increase the risk for heart disease and many other illnesses, including diabetes, stroke, arthritis, breathing problems, and depression. Here's an example of just how dangerous being overweight is: it is now an established medical fact that smoking is deadly; but obesity decreases the life expectancy of adults just as much as smoking. It can dramatically affect your health, and if left unaddressed long enough, it will.

The causes of this epidemic of increasing obesity are complex, but experts point to poor nutrition and our increasingly sedentary lives as the primary culprits. Although scientists have recently found genes that appear related to appetite and obesity, exactly how genetics affects weight is still not well understood. There is also research showing that individuals metabolize nutrients at different rates, which may help to explain why some people seem to gain weight more easily than others.

Although most weight gain is just a result of eating too much and exercising too little, it is possible that a medical condition could be responsible. If you have noticed a marked increase in your weight or waistline over a short period of time, at least part of this may be due to an underlying medical condition in need of treatment. Clues that this may be the case include other recent changes in your health, such as severe fatigue, muscle weakness, or leg swelling. Although these underlying medical conditions are relatively rare causes of weight gain, you should see your doctor if you have these symptoms.

What the Guidelines Say

Most people have a sense of whether they are overweight. But how do you really know—and, if you are, how much? Scientists have created a measure called the Body Mass Index (BMI) that takes into account both how much you weigh and how tall you are and produces a single number that identifies where you stand on a scale between being underweight and severely obese. The scale is not perfect, but it can give you a general idea of where you stand. If your BMI number is lower than 18.5 you're considered underweight. A BMI above 25 puts you in the overweight category. The expert guidelines say your BMI should be between 19 and 24.9. That's the range doctors consider optimal. Here are the formal BMI classifications:

Body Mass Index Weight and Obesity Classifications	
Category	BMI (kg/m²)
underweight	less than 18.5
normal	18.5 to 24.9
overweight	25 to 29.9
obesity, class I	30 to 34.9
obesity, class II	35 to 39.9
obesity, class III	40 or over
Adapted from the National Institutes of Health Clinical Guidelines on the Identification, Evaluation, and Treatment of Overweight and Obesity in Adults	

How do you determine your own BMI? You can refer to the chart on page 64, for one. If the weight/height categories you find there don't correspond with your own weight and height, you can use the following formulas (but most people prefer to use the chart):

Body Mass Index Formulas	
Using Metric Units	**Using Non-Metric Units**
BMI = WEIGHT (KG)/HEIGHT (M)^2	BMI = [WEIGHT (LBS.)/HEIGHT (IN.)^2] × 703
Example: A person who weighs 78.93 kilograms and is 1.77 meters tall has a BMI of 25: weight (78.93)/height (1.77)^2 = 25	Example: A person who is 164 pounds and is 68 inches tall has a BMI of 25: [weight (164)/height (68)^2] × 703 = 25

The Weight-Loss Strategy That Works

As the problem of overweight and obesity has grown in the United States, so has the number of diets, fads, supplements, and drinks claiming to help people lose weight. Many are controversial; some are actually dangerous. Yet the "secret formula" for losing weight could hardly be simpler: consume less fuel (in the form of food) than your body burns (by your activities). Human beings—and all other living things, for that matter—burn fuel to stay alive. The more active you are, the more fuel your body needs. We measure that fuel in units called *calories*. Calories (scientists call them "kilocalories") come from the food you eat. Much evidence suggests that your body doesn't really care where the calories come from; proteins, carbohydrates, and fats all can be turned into fuel. A recent study compared a low-fat versus a low-carbohydrate weight-loss diet, and after one year there was little difference in the results. Nevertheless, there is a need for more study because there is no consensus about how a person should best split his or her consumption of carbohydrates, fats, and proteins. Some experts are saying that the low-carbohydrate diets cannot be dismissed. People need to find what works best for them—and the strong recommendation from the American Heart Association is that you should re-strict your consumption of saturated fats.

You gain weight when you consume more calories of food than your body uses, or "metabolizes." You lose weight when the balance is tipped, even only slightly, the other way. Not all foods pack the same caloric punch. Fats, for example, contain far more calories per gram of weight than other foods.

You can lose weight by eating less, even if you change nothing else about your life. But it's also true that you can lose weight by continuing to eat what you always have and simply increasing your physical activity level. Either way, you'll be burning more fuel than you consume, and fat (which essentially is a kind of reservoir of stored energy in your body) will get used up. At any one time, about one-quarter of adult men and almost half of adult women are trying to lose weight. Of course, each of us has certain inherited predis-positions for weight gain or loss, and the balance between energy intake and energy use varies from individual to individual. But doc-tors have found that the most successful approach to weight loss and weight maintenance is a combination of diet, exercise, and mo-tivational strategies. Only after trying this first-line approach for at least six months should you and your doctor consider other ap-proaches to weight loss.

FEWER CALORIES Contrary to popular belief, losing weight doesn't simply mean eating less fat. It means eating fewer calories—of every kind. Your goal should be to lower, in a balanced manner, the total number of calories you consume in a given day *from all sources*. That's one reason why it's important to read nutri-tion labels on the food you buy: so you know not just how many calories they include, but also where those calories come from.

How much should you cut your calorie intake? The American Heart Association recommends that to lose weight, women should eat at least 1,200 and up to 1,500 calories per day and men should eat at least 1,500 and up to 1,800 calories per day. Most people are typically consuming well over 2,000, and often over 3,000 calories, each day. Therefore, it is a good idea to cut back gradually.

Calorie Counting		
Your weight (in pounds)	Calories You Use Per Day If You Are Moderately Active	Calories You Use Per Day If You Are Less Active
110	1,650	1,430
120	1,800	1,560
130	1,950	1,690
140	2,100	1,820
150	2,250	1,950
160	2,400	2,080
170	2,550	2,210
180	2,700	2,340
190	2,850	2,470
200	3,000	2,600
210	3,150	2,730
220	3,300	2,860
230	3,450	2,990
240	3,600	3,120
250	3,750	3,250
260	3,900	3,380
270	4,050	3,510
280	4,200	3,640
290	4,350	3,770
300	4,500	3,900

The key is to remember how many calories your body *actually* needs so that you can aim to consume a total number of calories that is lower than or up to your daily need. How many calories you need depends upon your current weight, your current level of physical activity, and—importantly—your own specific health needs. That's why you should work out your weight-loss program with your doctor. To start, you can get a general idea of how many calories you need each day by multiplying your weight (in pounds) by 15. This represents the average number of calories used in one day if you're moderately active. If you get very little exercise, multiply your weight by 13 instead of 15. (Less-active people burn fewer calories.) You can use the table on the previous page for reference. These numbers may actually overestimate daily calorie needs, but they can provide a useful reference point for most people.

According to the American Heart Association, here's what your diet should contain:

- no more than 5 to 8 teaspoons of fats and oils per day, including the fats used in cooking and baking and in salad dressings and spreads;

- 6 ounces or less of lean meat, fish, or skinless poultry daily; and

- no more than 3 or 4 egg yolks per *week*;

- 2 to 4 servings of nonfat or low-fat dairy products daily; and

- at least 5 servings of fruits and vegetables per day.

But the American Heart Association and the National Institutes of Health have also looked hard at the amounts and types of fats in our diet (and of sodium as well) and concluded the following:

- total fat intake should be less than 30% of total calorie intake;

- saturated fatty acid intake should be less than 10% of total calorie intake;

- polyunsaturated fatty acid intake should be no more than 10% of total calorie intake;

- monounsaturated fatty acid intake should make up the rest of total fat intake, about 10–15% of total calorie intake;

- cholesterol intake should be 300 mg per day at most; and

- sodium intake should be 3 g per day at most. and

For an explanation of the role of these different types of fats, and for information on diet programs that are effective for weight loss as well as heart health, turn to Chapter 3 ("Beyond the Key Strategies"), which also discusses many of the popular approaches to weight loss.

MORE EXERCISE   While exercise alone can reduce total body fat, it is actually not as effective as diet at reducing weight overall. On the other hand, when you combine diet and exercise you lose more weight, and do so more quickly, than if all you do is diet. What's more, exercising regularly helps keep you from regaining the weight you've lost—and that "rebound" weight gain is probably the most disheartening thing that happens to people who only diet. And, of course, exercise increases your cardiovascular fitness and is good for your heart in all the ways mentioned in Strategy #3.

For weight management, the National Institutes of Health guidelines recommend that you start off by walking for 30 minutes per day, 3 days per week, and then gradually build up to 45 minutes of intense walking for at least 5 days per week, and preferably every day. This regimen will help you burn an estimated 100 to 200 calories per day or more, improve your overall health, and strengthen your heart.

By the way, a recent study showed that you don't have to enroll in a formal exercise program; you can get the same benefits simply by increasing the level of physical activity in your daily routine (for example, taking the stairs instead of the elevator, or walking instead of driving).

A SUPPORT SYSTEM   The key to success in losing excess weight is staying motivated. But that's easier said than done.

Progress will be slow. How do you stay motivated? By monitoring your progress, managing stress, avoiding other triggers that make you want to eat, and getting friends and family to help. You may want to talk to your doctor or a nutritionist about the motivational strategies that can help you get the most out of your weight-management plan.

Research has demonstrated that this approach works. People who combine a low-calorie diet and exercise with behavioral therapy can expect to lose 5 to 10 percent of their starting weight over the course of four to six months. This level of weight loss is usually enough to improve many obesity-related conditions. Sometimes, however, it isn't enough.

Stronger Measures: Medication and Surgery

In more extreme cases of obesity, doctors may turn to prescription drugs and even surgery, especially if their patient's obesity is associated with other life-threatening health conditions. What's an extreme case? The National Institutes of Health recommend the use of prescription medications for weight loss only for people who have tried nondrug strategies without success. If you have a BMI of at least 30 or a BMI of at least 27 along with other obesity-related medical conditions, your doctor may recommend medications, typically as an addition to diet, exercise, and behavioral therapy. The drugs the Food and Drug Administration has approved for weight loss fall into two categories: those that suppress your appetite and those that reduce your digestive system's ability to absorb nutrients. There are many drugs in the first category, but some are approved only for short-term use, and most have relatively limited weight-loss effect, and so are not strongly recommended for patients with heart disease, high blood pressure, or advanced cardiovascular disease. A review of one of these drugs, sibutramine (trade name: Meridia) revealed that it is effective in promoting weight loss but had mixed effects on cardiovascular risk factors. There was no direct evidence that treatment with sibutramine improved health outcomes. The only FDA-approved drug in the second category is orlistat (trade name: Xenical). It cannot be used by patients who have digestive problems such as pancreatitis or a gallbladder condition called cholestasis, nor can it be taken by patients who are also taking cyclosporine, a medication often given after organ transplants. Otherwise, however, it is safe for people with heart disease to take this drug. Diarrhea is an occasional side effect.

Recently, researchers have found that certain drugs prescribed for epilepsy and migraine headaches also significantly reduce the weight of those taking them. They may alter the brain circuits that signal hunger and fullness. But these drugs have received little clinical research and, although some doctors are prescribing them for weight loss, they are not approved by the FDA for that purpose. Another drug that is under testing, rimonabant, has had a promising start. In a study presented at the annual meeting of the American College of Cardiology, investigators randomized 1,036 overweight or obese patients to placebo, 5 mg rimonabant, or 20 mg rimonabant for one year. Patients in the 20 mg group lost 15 pounds more than patients on placebo, and also experienced improvements in waist circumference, HDL, triglycerides, and many other markers of risk. This drug is also not yet approved by the FDA. Several other drugs are also under study.

Surgical procedures to reduce excess weight are used rarely. The clinical guidelines reserve the use of surgery for severely obese patients—that is, for those with a BMI of at least 40, or a BMI of at least 35 combined with obesity-related medical complications—and even then, only after they fail to respond sufficiently to medication. Obesity surgery (you may hear it called by its medical name, "bariatric surgery") reduces the size of the stomach. This surgery, which is receiving a lot of attention, makes a person feel full sooner and also reduces the desire for high-carbohydrate foods. Patients who undergo this kind of surgery may eventually lose 50 to 60 percent of their excess weight, and may also see a reversal of other obesity-related medical problems. But this surgical procedure is a radical last option; it necessitates a permanent change in lifestyle and diet and is still unsuccessful in one out of every five cases. In addition, it may require more than one surgery and may result in anemia. Nevertheless, for some people it may be the best option.

Frequently Asked Questions

Q: WHAT ABOUT DIETARY SUPPLEMENTS AND HERBAL PREPARATIONS?

There have been many over-the-counter supplements and remedies that claim to help with weight loss, including: chitosan, chromium picolinate, conjugate linoleic acid, ephedra alkaloids ("ma huang"), and garcinia cambogia. There is little research to demonstrate that any of these supplements are effective. Some of the most popular of these alternative medications contained ephedra, which is now banned by the FDA. The expert guidelines do not recommend any of the over-the-counter medications. If the combination of dietary changes, exercise, and behavior therapy has failed to bring your weight into normal and safe ranges, you should talk with your doctor about the option of taking medications that are well researched and specifically approved for the treatment of overweight and obesity.

Q: HOW QUICKLY CAN I EXPECT TO LOSE WEIGHT?

According to weight-management experts at the National Institutes of Health, your initial goal should be to lose 10 percent of your starting weight. A reasonable time for losing this first 10 percent is anywhere from three to twelve months. For instance, if your BMI is between 27 and 35, cutting down your calorie intake by 300 to 500 calories per day should result in a weight loss of about 0.5 to 1 pound per week. If your BMI is over 35, cutting down your calorie intake by 500 to 1,000 calories per day will lead to a weight loss of about 1 to 2 pounds per week. Both of these approaches work out to a 10 percent weight loss over approximately six months. Losing weight more quickly than this makes you more likely to regain the weight, since such rapid loss usually occurs through drastic—and unsustainable— changes to your diet or lifestyle. Worse, rapid weight loss can cause other health problems, such as gallbladder stones.

Q: DO THE GUIDELINES FOR LOSING WEIGHT APPLY TO OLDER ADULTS?

Because the research is limited in this group, the guidelines are currently not very specific about recommending weight loss in older people. There is some evidence to suggest that age alone should not prevent treatment of obesity. Other evidence suggests that being mildly overweight is not a risk factor for heart disease in the elderly and therefore weight reduction is not needed in such cases. One concern is that older people may be more sensitive than younger adults to overall reduced nutritional intake. There is also a higher risk in older adults that participation in a weight-loss program may mask weight loss that is actually caused by an underlying illness. Therefore, the experts recommend a careful assessment of the benefits and risks of weight loss for anybody age sixty-five or older. Weight loss in this group needs to be monitored carefully.

Q: WHAT ABOUT COMMERCIAL WEIGHT-LOSS PROGRAMS AND DIETS?

There are hundreds of heavily promoted commercial diets and weight-loss programs. The best programs are based on strong nutritional principles and do not promise to be either quick or easy. Many, of course, promise exactly that and, since such results can be achieved only through drastic action (if at all), are not based on sound nutritional principles. That means two things. First, they may be harmful to you. Second, there's little chance you'll be able to keep off the weight you lose. If you are considering a commercial weight-loss program, talk it over with a doctor and/or nutritionist first. You will want to choose a program based on sound principles and one that makes realistic claims about what it can help you achieve.

Q: WHAT ABOUT LOW-CARBOHYDRATE DIETS?

Diet fads come and go. The latest is the "low-carb" diet, which emphasizes cutting—in some cases even eliminating—the breads, pastas, rice, and other carbohydrates you consume. It's actually true that most Americans consume cabohydrates in excess. A low-carbohydrate diet may ultimately be proven safe and effective, but currently its benefits are being debated. A recent review of all the published studies of low-carbohydrate diets found that the evidence supporting the claims of these diets is weak, primarily because very few rigorous studies have been conducted on low-carb

Body Mass Index Chart

You can use this chart to match your height with your weight and then follow that column down to determine your body mass index (BMI). If your height or weight are not in this chart, you can use the formula on page 55 to calculate your BMI.

Find your height

Find the weight below that is closest to yours (in pounds)

Height (in feet and inches)	19	20	21	22	23	24	25	26	27	28	29	30	35	40
4' 10"	91	96	100	105	110	115	119	124	129	134	138	143	167	191
4' 11"	94	99	104	109	114	119	124	128	133	138	143	148	173	198
5'	97	102	107	112	118	123	128	133	138	143	148	153	179	204
5' 1"	100	106	111	116	122	127	132	137	143	148	153	158	185	211
5' 2"	104	109	115	120	126	131	136	142	147	153	158	164	191	218
5' 3"	107	113	118	124	130	135	141	146	152	158	163	169	197	225
5' 4"	110	116	122	128	134	140	145	151	157	163	169	174	204	232
5' 5"	114	120	126	132	138	144	150	156	162	168	174	180	210	240
5' 6"	118	124	130	136	142	148	155	161	167	173	179	186	216	247
5' 7"	121	127	134	140	146	153	159	166	172	178	185	191	223	255
5' 8"	125	131	138	144	151	158	164	171	177	184	190	197	230	262
5' 9"	128	135	142	149	155	162	169	176	182	189	196	203	236	270
5' 10"	132	139	146	153	160	167	174	181	188	195	202	207	243	278
5' 11"	136	143	150	157	165	172	179	186	193	200	208	215	250	286
6'	140	147	154	162	169	177	184	191	199	206	213	221	258	294
6' 1"	144	151	159	166	174	182	189	197	204	212	219	227	265	302
6' 2"	148	155	163	171	179	186	194	202	210	218	225	233	272	311
6' 3"	152	160	168	176	184	192	200	208	216	224	232	240	279	319
6' 4"	156	164	172	180	189	197	205	213	221	230	238	246	287	328
BMI (kg/m²)	19	20	21	22	23	24	25	26	27	28	29	30	35	40

diets, and most of those studies were of short duration. The primary finding was that weight loss in these studies appeared to be more related to calories than to carbohydrate content. The good news is that the studies did not indicate that the diet was harmful, though the long-term effects could not be assessed. So, despite the enthusiasm of advocates for this diet and recent small trials suggesting that low-carb diets have a lot of promise, the medical jury is still out. Currently, the nutrition experts who create the American Heart Association's dietary standards don't endorse it. And as a practical matter, the truth is that carbohydrates are a valuable and easily affordable source of energy. Eliminating them entirely from your diet means you'll have to get the calories you need from other sources—sources that may not be good for your overall health, such as fats. And for people over age sixty-five, whose nutrition may already be compromised, a low-carb diet may be quite harmful. If you choose to pursue a low-carbohydrate diet, you should ensure that you get adequate vitamins and minerals in the foods that you do eat. You should also check your cholesterol since the increase in fat intake may affect your levels. It is best *not* to feel free to indulge in eating as much fat as you would like. The bottom line is that you need to find what works best for you.

Strategy #5:
★★★ Take Charge of Your Blood Sugar

The primary fuel your body runs on is a form of sugar called *glucose*. Virtually everything you eat—proteins, carbohydrates, fats—eventually gets converted by your digestive system to this sugar compound. As is the case with so many of the delicate balances at work in the human body, you need to have enough glucose in your bloodstream to remain healthy, but if you have too much it can adversely affect your health. Precisely how much glucose gets absorbed from your bloodstream by the cells in your body at any given moment is regulated by a hormone called *insulin* that's produced by the pancreas. It helps to think of insulin as a key that unlocks a sort of gate in the walls of every cell through which the glucose passes to provide energy to the cell. When this system malfunctions—that is, when insulin is not succeeding in helping your cells absorb glucose—the cells become starved for energy and you begin to feel weak, tired, hungry, and often irritable. At the same time, because it's not getting to the cells, the sugar level rises in your bloodstream. This condition is called *diabetes*.

More than 10 million Americans are suffering from diagnosed diabetes. Another 5 million have the disease and don't know it. It's a condition that, if poorly controlled, damages blood vessels and eventually can cause a wide range of other problems. Damage to smaller blood vessels can and often does harm your eyes, kidneys, and nerves. Damage to larger blood vessels can lead to heart disease and high blood pressure. Diabetes can also cause impotence in men and increase the risk of infections of all kinds.

Until as recently as the 1920s, the "sugar disease," as it was long known, was inevitably fatal. Their bodies starved for energy, patients with the disease slipped into a coma and quickly died. Then, in 1921 a Canadian researcher, Fred Banting, and his student assistant, Charles Best, extracted insulin from a pancreas and injected it into ten diabetic dogs, saving their lives. Subsequent human experiments were equally successful. Their discovery led to a Nobel Prize for Banting (many think that Best also deserved it) and made it possible for diabetics to live long and productive lives.

Since then, scientists have identified two kinds of diabetes. In the case of Type I diabetes, the problem is that the pancreas doesn't produce enough insulin to let the glucose pass into the body's cells. This form of diabetes is typically inherited, usually appears in people at a young age, and is relatively uncommon. Insulin injections, to augment what the pancreas is producing, are the treatment for Type I diabetes.

In Type II diabetes, it's not that the body isn't producing enough insulin, it's that the cell walls have become resistant to it and therefore don't absorb the glucose they need. Type II diabetes typically appears later in life and is far more common than Type I; in fact, 90 percent of the people who are diagnosed with diabetes have the Type II form. Typically, this kind of diabetes is treated with drugs that cause the pancreas to create extra insulin to supply those cells that have not yet become resistant or by increasing the sensitivity of cells to insulin. But over a long enough time the pancreas can get overworked and these patients, too, may require insulin injections.

Researchers are not yet certain about what causes Type II diabetes, but it seems clear that, as with Type I, there is a strong genetic connection. That is, if someone in your family has had Type II diabetes, there is a greater likelihood that you will, too. Yet it is also increasingly clear that dietary and lifestyle choices play a significant role.

People who are overweight or obese have a much higher likelihood of developing Type II diabetes than people who are not. Unhealthy eating not only contributes to weight gain, but it also can put a much greater strain on your blood sugar/insulin balance. Overeating, especially eating a lot of simple carbohydrates (sweets, sweetened foods and drinks, chips, fries, and the like) that the body converts quickly to sugar, overloads the bloodstream with glucose, puts a strain on the insulin-production system, and appears to be connected to the development of insulin resistance. Chronic high blood sugar levels exact a significant toll on many parts of the body. They can cause loss of eyesight, kidney damage, and nerve disease, among other things.

There is a third blood sugar condition called "borderline" high glucose, or "impaired glucose tolerance," in which glucose remains in the bloodstream longer than is the case with people with normal glucose/insulin function. Researchers suspect that people with borderline high glucose already have developed some insulin resistance in their cell walls but have not yet reached the level of Type II diabetes. But that doesn't mean it's not a serious condition; borderline high glucose often develops into diabetes.

Testing for High Blood Sugar

How do you know whether your blood sugar levels are too high? A simple series of blood tests will tell you. To be certain the results are reliable, these tests typically are done on two separate occasions. You are diabetic if:

- your "fasting blood glucose" level is at least 126 mg/dL;

- you have a blood glucose level of at least 200 mg/dL two hours after a meal; or

- you have a random blood glucose level of at least 200 mg/dL *and* have symptoms such as excess thirst and frequent urination.

What the Guidelines Say

The American Diabetes Association guidelines say that *if you do not yet have diabetes* you should have your blood glucose levels checked at least every three years starting at age forty-five. But you should have it checked even more frequently if any of the following apply to you:

- you have any disease of the blood vessels, such as heart disease, stroke, or atherosclerosis;

- your body mass index (BMI) is 25 or greater;

- your blood pressure is higher than 140/90;

- your HDL (good) cholesterol measures 35 mg/dL or less;

- you have a triglyceride level of 250 mg/dL or more;

- you have parents or siblings with diabetes;

- you have been told at any time in the past that you have "borderline" high blood sugar;

- you are habitually inactive;

- you are a member of an ethnic group with a high risk for diabetes (African-American, Hispanic-American, Native American, Asian-American, or Pacific Islander);

- you are a woman who has delivered a baby of more than nine pounds or has been diagnosed with gestational diabetes; or

- you have been diagnosed with polycystic ovarian syndrome.

On the other hand, *if you do have diabetes already* the guidelines urge you to have your blood glucose tested every three months, or even more often depending upon the type and severity of the diabetes you have, what treatments you are receiving, and how well the disease is being controlled.

In addition, your doctor should be ordering a "hemoglobin A1c (HbA1c) level" test for you (also called glycosylated hemoglobin). Hemoglobin is a molecule that exists in red blood cells and carries oxygen. HbA1c forms when excess blood sugar attaches to the hemoglobin in those cells. The more glucose in your bloodstream, the more HbA1c will be present. And because HbA1c stays in your bloodstream for a long time, this test makes it possible for your doctor to get a kind of overall average of the glucose that's been in your bloodstream during the past three months, not just the past day or two. This not only provides a more reliable indication of your long-term condition but also makes it possible for the doctor to know whether you have been following your treatment program regularly or have simply fasted the day before your blood glucose test to get a good result—a not uncommon practice. To stay healthy, you need to keep the HbA1c level in your bloodstream below 7 percent. You should know your sugar test results. In Appendix B, there is a tool to help you do that.

Blood Sugar and Your Heart

Why do we focus on diabetes in a book about heart disease? Because people with diabetes have an especially high risk of developing heart disease. If they do get heart disease, their heart problems tend to be worse than those in people without diabetes. In addition, people with diabetes have five times the risk of having a heart attack that non-diabetics do.

In fact, research has shown that simply having an elevated

blood sugar level—even without diabetes—is a risk for heart disease. A large United Kingdom study involving more than 5,000 people with diabetes found that for every 1 percent reduction of HbA1c, there was an 18 percent reduction in heart attacks and a 25 percent reduction in all diabetes-related deaths. The reasons are fairly simple. First, people with diabetes often have high LDL (bad) cholesterol levels and low HDL (good) cholesterol levels, both of which lead to faster rates of atherosclerosis. Second, they also tend to have high blood pressure, in part because they are overweight. Third, they have a greater tendency to form blood clots. And finally, they have a higher likelihood of inflammation in the blood, which is closely linked to increased heart disease risk.

Strategies for Controlling Blood Sugar

If you have heart disease, it's critical to control your blood sugar levels. It's that simple because the link between high blood sugar and more severe heart problems is that clear. The good news is that even if you have what's known as "borderline high" blood glucose levels, are overweight or obese, or have a family history of the disease, you can prevent yourself from developing Type II diabetes. And if you already have it, you can control it. Oddly enough, the strategies for getting your blood sugar levels under control, or keeping them under control, are the same as the strategies we've seen in other sections of this book: diet, weight control, and exercise—and if those are not sufficient, medications.

DIET   It was once thought that people with diabetes should avoid eating anything sugary, but there was never any scientific evidence to support this conclusion. Since almost everything you eat eventually is converted to sugar (glucose) anyway, what matters most is that you regulate the number of calories you eat. Eating a large quantity of a simple carbohydrate, such as potatoes, bread, or rice, can indeed quickly load your bloodstream with glucose. The answer for most people isn't to stop eating such foods, but to control how much of them you eat. How much is too much? That's something you and your doctor will work out based upon your glucose tests. But as a general rule, the American Diabetes Association says simply that you should maintain a diet that is low in calories, low in fats, and well balanced nutritionally. Still crave something sweet? Artificial sweeteners can help make a fine substitute.

These basic nutritional guidelines will reduce your blood sugar to acceptable levels if you follow them closely. Some nutritionists and doctors nonetheless believe you should limit your intake of foods with what is known as a high "glycemic index"—that is, foods that will rapidly increase sugar levels in your body after you eat them.

The glycemic index is a relative scale of how fast circulating blood sugar rises after the consumption of a certain carbohydrate. The top of the scale is 100, which is the value for glucose itself. The glycemic load is a measure of the full impact of the carbohydrate, taking the glycemic index into account. The glycemic load is the glycemic index divided by 100 and multiplied by the available carbohydrate content (carbohydrate minus fiber) in grams. A glycemic load of 20 or more is considered high.

Here are some examples:

Food	Glycemic Index	Glycemic Load (per serving)
instant rice	91	24.8 (110 g)
baked potato	85	20.3 (110 g)
corn flakes	84	21.0 (225 mL)
carrot	71	3.8 (55 g)
white bread	70	21.0 (2 slices)
rye bread	65	19.5 (2 slices)
muesli	56	16.8 (110 mL)
banana	53	13.3 (170 g)
spaghetti	41	16.4 (55 g)
apple	36	8.1 (170 g)
lentil beans	29	5.7 (110 mL)
milk	27	3.2 (225 mL)
peanuts	14	0.7 (30 g)

There is some obvious logic to this approach; after all, consuming quantities of these foods simply makes it harder to control your blood sugar levels. But the long-term effects of following a diet based on the glycemic index are still unclear and consequently the American Diabetes Association guidelines do not currently endorse using the glycemic index. However, research in this area is growing, and many doctors and patients, betting that future studies will show benefits of using the glycemic index, are tailoring their diets accordingly.

WEIGHT   Being obese or overweight, especially if that weight consists significantly of abdominal body fat, is closely linked to insulin resistance. That's the bad news. The good news is that research shows that losing this weight lowers that insulin resistance. Moderate weight loss, on the scale of 10 to 20 pounds, has been shown to lead to lower glucose levels, cholesterol, and blood pressure—all outcomes that reduce your risk of heart disease. Of course, losing weight and keeping it off is seldom easy. For how to do it successfully, review the preceding section, Strategy #4: Take Charge of Your Weight.

EXERCISE   For people with high glucose levels, exercise alone can have a remarkable effect. For reasons that are not entirely clear, it appears that regular exercise can reduce insulin resistance in cells, increase glucose absorption, and, as a result, decrease glucose levels in the bloodstream. This effect works best for people who have good glucose control and are taking oral anti-diabetic medications, but the benefits of exercise for all people with diabetes or borderline high glucose are clear. An analysis of multiple studies shows that regular exercise training over the long term can lower HbA1c levels close to 1 percent, regardless of what diabetic treatment the patient is following. Studies also show that people with diabetes who exercise at least two hours per week have a 40 percent lower risk of heart disease or stroke. Of course some people with diabetes have conditions that limit their ability to exercise (blood vessel disease, loss of circulation or sensation in the feet, heart disease), so you should ask your doctor what kind of exercise program would best suit your needs. Refer to Strategy #3: Take Charge of Your Fitness.

Controlling Blood Sugar with Medication

If diet, weight loss, and exercise fail to bring your blood glucose levels within the normal range, your doctor will prescribe either oral anti-diabetic medications, insulin injections, or some combination of the two.

ORAL ANTI-DIABETIC MEDICATION   Most people who have not been able to bring their blood sugar under control by lifestyle changes begin with oral medication. There are a number of such medications, and a large number of clinical trials have proven them effective in many cases. However, each class of the medication works differently and has different possible side effects. The most common of these effects is *hypoglycemia*, a condition in which blood sugar drops too low and leaves the patient weak, light-headed, and even faint. It may take a bit of trial and error for you and your doctor to find the medication, or combination of medications, that works best in your particular case and has the least unpleasant side effects. The choices are described below.

INSULIN   Oral anti-diabetic drugs work by encouraging the pancreas to produce more insulin than it normally does. That's why, for example, oral medications typically don't help patients with Type I diabetes, whose pancreases are unable to produce insulin at all. But even in Type II diabetics these medications can effectively overwork and wear out the patient's pancreas, so that it ends up producing very little or no insulin on its own. When that happens, injections of insulin are needed to replace what the pancreas can no longer make. Although the daily task of taking regular insulin injections and timing them with your meals is not as easy as taking a few pills, a properly designed insulin regimen can be much more effective at controlling glucose levels for many people. Apart from inconvenience, the primary side effect for most people is modest weight gain.

Oral Anti-Diabetic Medications	
sulfonylureas (glyburide, glimepiride, glipizide)	Sulfonylureas act quickly and are very effective at lowering blood glucose levels. However, they are prone to cause hypoglycemia.
short-acting secretagogues (repaglinide, nateglinide)	Short-acting secretagogues are often best taken before meals because they are very rapid- and short-acting. These medications may also cause hypoglycemia.
alpha-glucosidase inhibitors (acarbose, miglitol)	Alpha-glucosidases are designed to reduce the amount of food absorbed by your body with each meal. However, their effect on decreasing HbA1c is small, and they can often cause diarrhea, bloating, and gas.
metformin	Often prescribed as a first-line medication, metformin has been used for years and is very effective for controlling glucose levels. Metformin can lower insulin resistance while limiting weight gain. It also does not tend to cause hypoglycemia. However, metformin should not be used by people with kidney failure, heart failure, or liver disease.
"glitazones" (pioglitazone, rosiglitazone)	These new medications help to control blood glucose by lowering insulin resistance. The glitazones also help to lower cholesterol levels. However, glitazones need to be taken for weeks before any benefit is seen, and they can cause swelling and weight gain as side effects. They should be used with caution in people with heart failure.

INSULIN PLUS ORAL MEDICATIONS It used to be thought that once patients reached the stage of needing insulin injections they no longer needed to take oral anti-diabetic medications. But new research has demonstrated that combining insulin injections and an oral medication may actually be more effective at helping people control their glucose levels. Taking both, it turns out, reduces the amount of insulin they need to inject and helps balance glucose levels over the course of the day. However, since insulin combined with some oral medications, such as rosiglitazone and pioglitazone, may increase the risk of fluid retention and possibly heart failure, you should be monitored closely if you take these medications.

Frequently Asked Questions

Q: IF I HAVE DIABETES, WHAT OTHER KINDS OF HEALTH CHECKS SHOULD I HAVE?

In addition to contributing to heart disease, poorly controlled diabetes can compromise other critical systems in your body, and it's important to keep track of their condition. For example, you should have your urine checked for protein at the time you are diagnosed with diabetes and at least once a year afterward to determine whether you have any kidney damage. Also, you should have your eyes examined by an ophthalmologist or optometrist trained to screen for diabetic eye disease soon after you are diagnosed with diabetes, and then once a year afterward. Your feet should be inspected at every routine doctor's visit, and you should have a complete foot examination at least once a year because a combination of circulatory and nerve damage can make them susceptible to infection and ulceration. To guard against infections, you should receive an annual flu shot and a vaccination against pneumonia at least once in your lifetime.

Q: WHAT IS "TIGHT" GLUCOSE CONTROL?

People with diabetes who are able to keep their glucose levels within the normal or target range over a long period of time are much less likely to develop complications. "Tight" glucose control means adhering closely to the following glucose levels:

- blood glucose between 90 and 130 mg/dL before meals;

- blood glucose below 180 mg/dL after meals; and

- HbA1c less than 7% at regular checks every 2 to 3 months.

Controlling your glucose levels this tightly is hard work and requires careful diet planning, the right medications, diligence, and a lot of patience. But by partnering with your doctor to achieve this level of control, and by getting the support of friends and family to sustain it, you will not only feel better, but stay healthier over the long term.

Q: I'VE BEEN DIAGNOSED WITH DIABETES. WILL I HAVE IT FOR THE REST OF MY LIFE?

Not necessarily. It's true that for most people having diabetes is like having heart disease: it is a chronic condition for which doctors have yet to find a cure. But some people with Type II diabetes have been able to cure themselves of the disease by losing weight, exercising, and changing their diet. Insulin resistance, the cause of Type II diabetes, is associated with excess body fat. Decreasing this fat can decrease insulin resistance and, for some people, effectively cure their diabetes. In rare cases, well-controlled Type II diabetes may even resolve on its own, without much weight loss. In all of these cases, however, patients must maintain the healthy lifestyle that brought about these changes and be vigilant about the possibility of their diabetes returning.

Q: WHAT ABOUT PANCREAS TRANSPLANTS?

Complete pancreas transplants are possible, but typically they are limited to patients with Type I diabetes who have severe kidney disease or for whom insulin therapy has been unsuccessful, resulting in major illness. Researchers are also investigating the possible benefit of transplanting the pancreatic cells that make insulin, called "islet cells," from another healthy pancreas, instead of transplanting an entire pancreas. But pancreatic islet cell transplants are still in the experimental phase and probably will not be available for a number of years.

Q: DOES TAKING INSULIN CAUSE WEIGHT GAIN?

Technically, yes. People who begin to take either oral medications or insulin may gain a few extra pounds: two to six pounds in the case of oral medications and as much as nine pounds in the case of insulin therapy. Most of this weight gain occurs during the first three to five years of treatment and is thought to be simply the regaining of weight originally lost as a result of having untreated diabetes. This weight gain is small and poses no significant health risk, especially when compared with the immense benefit gained from treating the diabetes and achieving tight glucose control. What's more, new research suggests that using combination therapy (oral medication plus insulin) may result in less weight gain than using insulin alone.

Strategy #6:
★★★ Take Charge of Your Smoking

After decades of willful misinformation by tobacco companies, the world now knows what doctors have long warned: smoking is lethal. It is the number-one cause of avoidable illness and death in the nation, killing almost a half-million people every year. If smoking were a disease, it would be considered an epidemic of epic proportions. And lung cancer isn't the only cause of these deaths; smoking causes or severely worsens a wide range of medical conditions, including other forms of cancer, obstructive lung disease, stroke, pregnancy complications, and—most important to us—heart disease.

Smoking and Your Heart

How does smoking cause heart disease? Researchers have demonstrated conclusively that atherosclerotic plaques build up in the arteries 50 percent faster in smokers than in non-smokers. What's more, nicotine itself causes heart problems: it triggers the release of high amounts of adrenaline in the body, which, in turn, increases blood pressure. It turns out you don't even have to be a smoker to develop heart problems; all you have to do is live with one: secondhand smoke increases a person's risk of heart problems by up to 60 percent. If you've already had a heart attack and continue to smoke, you have a 50 percent higher risk for having another heart problem than non-smokers do.

On the other hand, if you do quit smoking after that heart attack, your risk for future heart problems falls to the same level as that of non-smokers within three years of quitting. That's not the only benefit. After your last cigarette:

- your blood pressure goes down to what it was before you started smoking within twenty minutes;

- the level of carbon monoxide in your blood drops within hours;

- your lung function improves by 30 percent in two to three months;

- your risk for heart disease drops by 50 percent within one year; and

- your risk of stroke decreases to the level of a non-smoker within five to fifteen years.

What the Guidelines Say

The American Heart Association/American College of Cardiology guidelines couldn't be clearer: If you smoke, stop. And avoid being exposed to secondhand smoke as well.

Mark Twain once said, "To cease smoking is the easiest thing I ever did. I ought to know because I've done it a thousand times." Some 50 million people in America smoke, and seven out of every ten of them have tried to quit at least once. Fewer than 20 percent of these people are still smoke-free one year later. Why? Because smoking isn't a bad habit; it's an addiction.

The tars and other substances in tobacco are what cause lung cancer and other diseases, but it's the nicotine in the leaves that keeps you wanting more even though you know it's harming you. Nicotine, like alcohol, is both a stimulant and a relaxant. It stimulates the production of adrenaline (among other things that increase your heartbeat) but also affects neurotransmitter chemicals in your brain to produce a mild euphoria. It is very fast-acting; it takes only seven seconds for nicotine to reach your brain after you inhale cigarette smoke. But it also doesn't last long; its effect wanes in less than an hour. When that happens, your brain craves more. When it doesn't get it, you become irritable, anxious, and headachy. That's nicotine's addiction cycle.

Most people who smoke started in their teenage years. They may have experimented with cigarettes, drawn by the symbolic act of defiance. By age twenty, 80 percent of smokers regret that they started smoking. Unfortunately, the hold of the nicotine makes it difficult for them to quit.

You can cure a bad habit by willpower alone, but it takes serious work to kick an addiction. Some people can do it without help, but many more cannot. For the most part, people who fail when they try to stop smoking have failed only in understanding that for most people it takes a complex mix of medical and psychological strategies—and a lot of support from others—to kick this addiction for good. The expert guidelines recommend a combination of medications, organized smoking cessation programs, and counseling.

How to Stop Smoking

For something so difficult, the "prescription" to stop smoking successfully is simple:

- decide you want to quit;

- design a program for quitting with your doctor;

- get support from others;

- set a quit date; and . . .

- quit.

DECIDE YOU WANT TO QUIT The sheer difficulty of kicking an addiction, the discomfort, the fear of failure, the abandonment of familiar patterns of being and habits of acting—all these things and more make simply deciding to quit an enormous hurdle to overcome. Yet millions of people make that decision every year. The hard part is making it stick. As in so many things that are difficult in life, knowledge can help smooth the way. Let's begin with the positive: the rewards of quitting. You'll soon:

- become medically healthier;

- feel physically healthier;

- perform better in any physical activity;

- improve your self-esteem;

- enjoy a great sense of accomplishment;

- find that food tastes better;

- improve your sense of smell;

- improve the smell of your home, car, and clothing;

- find that your breath will be fresher;

- enhance your skin;

- know that you won't be exposing people around you to smoke;

- no longer have to worry about quitting; and

- save a lot of money.

That's a pretty impressive list of positives. Add to that list the fact that smoking is a powerful predictor of sudden death, increasing the risk of this tragic effect about twofold. But the good news is that the risk goes down when you quit.

If the benefits are so clear, why do people fail? Because it's hard; stopping smoking will present you with some very difficult challenges—at least in the beginning. You may:

- have to change your routine to avoid situations in which you typically smoked;

- miss the physical pleasures of smoking;

- feel depressed;

- experience unpleasant withdrawal symptoms;

- find that the fear of failure will be ever-present;

- gain weight; and

- have trouble asking for and getting enough support from friends and family.

Make your own list of the reasons you want to stop smoking. Write them down and put the list where you'll see it often. At the top of the list, write this: *Because I'll live longer and healthier, and I owe that to myself and to those who care about me.* Then see your doctor.

DESIGN A PROGRAM FOR QUITTING WITH YOUR DOCTOR

Because tobacco is both physiologically and psychologically addictive, you need help in addressing both kinds of addiction. That is, you'll need both medication and counseling.

The FDA has approved five medications to help people quit smoking, all of which are effective. Four of these medications are types of *nicotine-replacement therapy*: gum, inhalers, nasal sprays, and patches. Nicotine-replacement products reduce withdrawal symptoms but, unlike smoking, do not contain tar or other harmful toxins and are not as addictive. Although nicotine-replacement medications can be bought without a prescription, you should talk to your doctor before using them to find what will work best for you.

The fifth medication, the antidepressant bupropion (trade name: Zyban and Wellbutrin SR—the "SR" is for "sustained release"), causes somewhat less weight gain than other medications. When given with intensive behavioral support, bupropion is as effective as nicotine-replacement therapy and can nearly double your chance of quitting smoking. Prolonged use may be helpful in preventing relapse. Bupropion is contraindicated in patients with current or past epilepsy and in those at risk of seizure (e.g., alcohol abusers). It should also not be used for patients with severe liver disease or bipolar disorder.

Each of these alternatives has advantages and disadvantages, as laid out in the following table:

Smoking Cessation Medications: Pros and Cons	
bupropion SR	Many people like the convenience of this once-a-day pill. Others dislike the insomnia and dry mouth it can cause. It should not be taken by those with seizures, eating disorders, known allergy to the drug, or those taking monoamine oxidase inhibitor antidepressants.
nicotine gum	Many people like the ease and flexibility of using the gum. Others dislike the taste, having to use it frequently, or the jaw ache it can cause.
nicotine inhaler	Many people like the flexibility of using the inhaler and find that it feels similar to smoking. Others dislike having to use it frequently, or the mouth and throat discomfort that it can cause.
nicotine nasal spray	Many people like the flexibility of dosing. Others dislike having to use it frequently, or the nose and eye irritation that it can cause.
nicotine patch	Many people like the once-a-day use of the patch. Others prefer a more flexible medication or dislike the skin rash that it can occasionally cause.

Nicotine replacement and bupropion, alone or together, but in combination with a physician-patient partnership, may provide the best opportunity to success.

Another medication, called clonidine, also is effective, but because of potential side effects it should be used only when first-line medications have failed. Two other medication strategies have also been tried: the antidepressant nortriptyline, and the combined use of a nicotine patch along with another form of nicotine replacement. Relatively little research has been done on these treatment strategies.

Because addiction is both physical and mental, medication alone is unlikely to successfully help you stop smoking. Counseling, which is available from many different professionals—doctors, nurses, psychologists, social workers, even dentists and pharmacists—has proven to be essential to smokers who want to quit and stay smoke-free over the long term. Often the need for professional support when craving and other withdrawal symptoms hit is too immediate for appointment-scheduling with a counselor. Thankfully, there are many twenty-four-hour, toll-free "quitlines" staffed by counselors trained to help people quit smoking. Studies show that using a quitline may as much as double your chance of staying smoke-free after quitting. There are now quitlines in thirty-three states and a national quitline sponsored by the American Cancer Society. For more information, simply call the American Cancer Society at 1-800-ACS-2345.

In addition to these proven medication and counseling treatments, other forms of treatment have been promoted as effective but still need more research to confirm their usefulness. These treatments include hypnosis, gradually cutting down the number of cigarettes smoked, positive and negative physiological feedback techniques, individual and group 12-step programs, restricted environmental stimulation (a form of therapy that, among other things, fosters reflection on the reasons one smokes), a drug called mecamylamine, and antidepressants other than bupropion or nortriptyline. Also, rimonabant, the experimental drug that was found to be effective for weight loss, may have benefits for smoking cessation.

Finally, there are two treatments that have been tried in the past for which there is no convincing evidence of effectiveness: acupuncture and the ingestion of silver acetate.

GET SUPPORT FROM OTHERS People who smoke associate many of their daily activities—meals, a coffee break, or having a drink with friends, to name but a few—with having a cigarette. Their social interactions are strongly linked with smoking. Indeed as smoking has become banned in many places, smokers' own friendship patterns are affected, often limiting them to relationships with other smokers. All of these patterns and relationships make quitting more difficult, and in many instances succeeding will require a change in these patterns and the support of family and friends when you are tempted to light up again. This support is critical; researchers have found that people with ongoing social support are 50 percent more likely to be successful at quitting and staying smoke-free.

SET A QUIT DATE The next step is to set a date when you will stop smoking. This is actually more complicated than it sounds. Choose a day when you will be busy and be able to avoid places or social situations that you associate with smoking. For example, if you tend to smoke more at work or on weekdays, choose a Saturday or the beginning of a holiday. If you smoke more on the weekends, choose a Monday, or some other workday. In addition, choose a day when you will be able to take some time at the end to reward yourself in some fashion for having quit. Finally, tell your friends and family so that they can support you and help you celebrate.

As you approach your quit date, consider following the practical "Five-Day Plan to Get Ready to Quit Smoking" developed by the United States Surgeon General, on the next page.

Frequently Asked Questions

Q: HOW WILL I FEEL JUST AFTER I QUIT SMOKING?

Even if you are taking nicotine-replacement therapy, you may still experience withdrawal symptoms after you stop smoking. These include cravings for tobacco, irritability, restlessness, increased appetite, trouble concentrating, fatigue, anxiety, depression, consti-

Five-Day Plan to Get Ready to Quit Smoking	
5 days to Quit Day	List all of your reasons for quitting and tell your friends and family about your plan. Stop buying cartons of cigarettes.
4 days to Quit Day	Pay attention to when and why you smoke. Think of new ways to relax or things to hold in your hand instead of a cigarette. Think of habits or routines you may want to change. Make a list to use when you quit.
3 days to Quit Day	Make a list of the things you could do with the extra money you will save by not buying cigarettes. Think of who to reach out to when you need help, like a smoking support group.
2 days to Quit Day	Buy the over-the-counter nicotine patch or nicotine gum, or get a prescription for the nicotine inhaler, nasal spray, or the non-nicotine pill, bupropion SR. Clean your clothes to get rid of the smell of cigarette smoke.
1 day to Quit Day	Think of a reward you will get yourself after you quit. Make an appointment with your dentist to have your teeth cleaned. At the end of the day, throw away all cigarettes and matches. Put away lighters and ashtrays.
Quit Day	Keep very busy. Change your routine when possible, and do things out of the ordinary that don't remind you of smoking. Remind friends, family, and coworkers that this is your quit day, and ask them to help and support you. Avoid alcohol. Buy yourself a treat, or do something to celebrate.
1 day after Quit Day	Congratulate yourself. When cravings hit, do something that isn't connected with smoking, like taking a walk, drinking a glass of water, or taking some deep breaths. Call your support network. Find things to snack on, like carrots, sugarless gum, or air-popped popcorn.

pation, gas, and stomach upset. Each of these symptoms can be managed using the coping strategies described above.

Q: HOW CAN I AVOID THE URGE TO SMOKE?

You probably can't. But you can take steps to avoid places or situations that you connect with smoking, thus decreasing the frequency with which those urges arise. Also, avoid coffee, soft drinks, and alcohol, all of which can make your cravings worse.

Q: WHAT CAN I DO WHEN THE URGE TO SMOKE HITS?

Distract yourself. Sounds silly, doesn't it? But it works. Much of the urge to smoke comes from the association you make between the activities you're used to pursuing and smoking. Now when the craving hits, do something else right away: take a few deep breaths, drink some water, listen to music, talk to a friend, take a bath, go for a walk, or busy yourself with a task or chore. The craving will pass, as will the stress that comes along with it. Whatever you do, don't smoke. Not even one puff. It will only make your cravings worse.

Q: I'VE TRIED TO QUIT MANY TIMES BEFORE. NOW WHAT?

Don't be discouraged. People who have quit smoking usually have tried two or three or more times before managing to stay smoke-free. Try to identify what caused you to start smoking again in the past and think about how you'll deal with these challenges this time. By the same token, think about what helped you stay smoke-free in the past and try those strategies again. Also, ask friends or family to help you stay on track.

A PATIENT'S VIEW:
FINDING THE WILL TO QUIT

I had no idea that I had heart disease. I do a lot of heavy lifting in my work, and I always felt great. I just don't go to doctors for small things. I was forty-five years old and hadn't been to a doctor in more than twenty years. I never gave much thought to my health. For many years,

I drank beer at night, almost every night of the week. I smoked a pack of cigarettes or more every day for more than thirty years.

Then, one day I had chest pain that hurt so bad that I could barely walk. It would come and go, but was especially bad when I was carrying something. One day I couldn't even climb a ladder. I went to a doctor who told me that I had acid reflux disease and prescribed that purple pill. I went back and he started ordering a bunch of stomach tests. I have a buddy whose sister works at the hospital and she told me that I needed a stress test. When I finally had one, the diagnosis of heart disease was clear. I was hospitalized soon after that and had a stent placed to open the artery.

I knew that I needed to make some changes. I just about stopped drinking and started exercising. My cholesterol and blood pressure were high and I take medications to control them. I changed my diet so that I eat less fat and salt. As a result of these changes I lost almost thirty pounds.

The biggest thing by far was the smoking. I knew what I should do but I just could not get myself to do it. I remember clearly the day that I gained the strength to quit smoking. My niece was having a birthday and I offered to take her to the store to buy a present. She looked at me and said that all she wanted was for me to quit smoking. I laughed at first and asked her why. She replied that someday she was going to get married and she wanted me to be there. I was stunned. Those words hit me like a ton of bricks.

Quitting cigarettes was not easy. I started by leaving them at home and not smoking at work. The first weeks and months were awful. Some days I felt like I could kill someone for a cigarette. The withdrawal was hell. I actually don't quite remember how I did it. I just smoked fewer and fewer until I just was able to let them go. It took about four to six months for me to get over the difficult part.

The truth is that I do cheat sometimes. I have a life, and once a week or so I get together with some friends. We have a few drinks and I may have a cigarette or two. Once I leave that scene I am fine again and do not need them. After thirty years of smoking I think that's pretty good.

—Mike

Strategy #7:
★★★ Take Charge of Your Medications

You may have noticed something curious about the previous six strategies for taking charge of your heart disease: most of them don't involve taking drugs, at least not as the first line of treatment. For many of the key risk factors of heart disease—high blood pressure, cholesterol, excess weight, excess blood sugar (though not necessarily smoking)—the first steps are the same: diet, exercise, and weight control. Medications have a role if these first steps fail to bring the condition under control, but most doctors don't turn to them right at the outset of a treatment program.

But for heart disease itself, several medications are absolutely critical and can mean the difference between life and death—right from the beginning:

- aspirin and other so-called "blood thinners";

- beta-blockers;

- ACE inhibitors; and

- statins or other cholesterol-lowering medications for selected patients (described in Strategy #2).

Each of these drugs has different purposes. For example, aspirin and other blood thinners work to keep blood flowing through arteries clogged by heart disease. Beta-blockers and ACE inhibitors help those who have had a heart attack from having another. And there are other combinations of these drugs to suit specific conditions. Exactly what combination will work best for you is something you'll work out with your doctor, in part as a safeguard against negative drug interactions or allergic reactions. But if you have heart disease, these are drugs you will need to know about.

★★★ Aspirin and Other Blood Thinners
The ability of blood to clot is what keeps us from bleeding to death when we're cut and, conversely, what makes ordinary life dangerous

for people who have conditions that keep their blood from clotting. But in people with heart disease, clots can slow or stop the flow of blood in coronary arteries, starving the heart of oxygen and triggering heart attacks. That's why medicines that inhibit the ability of blood to clot—called "blood thinners"—are a key weapon in the battle against heart disease. Aspirin, highly effective and inexpensive, tops the list of blood-thinning drugs used for this purpose, but there are others as well.

Aspirin: The "New" Wonder Drug for Heart Disease.   Healers at least since the ancient Egyptians have known there was something in the bark of willow trees and wintergreen plants that reduced pain. Centuries later, the "something" was identified as salicylic acid. It was a remarkably effective pain-reliever and fever-reducer, but taken in its pure form it had some pretty nasty side effects—it caused nausea and severe stomach irritation. Scientists in a number of countries tried to formulate less toxic derivatives, but it wasn't until the late 1890s that a German chemist, whose father had rheumatoid arthritis, came up with a compound—*acetylsalicylic acid*—that worked without causing harm. The chemist worked for Bayer and Company, and they named the compound "aspirin." Labeled the "wonder drug," it has been the leading non-narcotic painkiller ever since.

It wasn't until quite recently, however, that researchers discovered that aspirin was also a wonder at preventing heart problems. During the past thirty years, roughly 150 studies have demonstrated repeatedly and conclusively that taking just a single aspirin tablet a day can reduce your risk of a heart attack by as much as 30 percent, and reduce your risk of having a stroke as well. And that's not all. Taking aspirin at the first sign of a heart attack greatly reduces your risk of complications and death. After bypass surgery, angioplasty, or stenting, aspirin helps keep arteries from becoming blocked again.

Indeed, aspirin protects more than just the heart. After bypass surgery, for example, it lowers the risk of stroke, kidney problems, and bowel problems; in addition, daily aspirin use is associated with a significantly lower risk of developing precancerous growths in the colon; and long-term use of aspirin or other anti-inflammatory medications may reduce the risk of Alzheimer's disease.

How Does It Work?   The truth is, we don't completely know. But a couple of things are clear. Aspirin is a "blood thinner." During the 1960s, researchers found that a dose of aspirin could inhibit the normal process by which platelets form clots. By keeping clots from forming, aspirin keeps blood flowing to the heart. More recently, researchers have begun to understand that inflammation of the arteries can also lead to heart disease. Aspirin calms inflammation and thus may also help to prevent heart disease in this way.

What Do the Guidelines Say?   The American Heart Association/American College of Cardiology guidelines are clear: take one aspirin tablet per day for the rest of your life. Unlike other medications, where different doses have different effects, studies show that any dose from 75 to 325 mg (the most common tablet strengths), taken once a day, will have about the same effect. If you've recently had a heart attack, you should take another medication, clopidogrel (discussed below) in addition to aspirin for at least nine months. If you can't tolerate aspirin's side effects, take clopidogrel or warfarin (discussed below) instead.

What Are Aspirin's Side Effects?   Aspirin is one of the safest drugs on the market today. That's why you can buy it "over the counter," without a prescription. Still, even aspirin can have side effects. It can damage the lining of the stomach and, occasionally, cause ulcers that can bleed. But these risks are fairly small; studies have shown that only one in a hundred people who take aspirin for two years will experience stomach or intestinal bleeding. If you've been taking aspirin and develop stomach pain, and especially if your stool turns black sometimes (indicating the presence of blood), you should stop taking it and contact your doctor.

In addition, because it inhibits clotting, aspirin sometimes can keep clots from forming in places where they're needed, increasing the tendency to bleed. This can cause minor problems, like an increased vulnerability to bruising, or serious problems, including a major hemorrhage. The most catastrophic complication may be bleeding that occurs in the brain, a condition called hemorrhagic stroke. But this condition is very rare. Research has demonstrated that only one in 1,000 people who take aspirin for three years will be affected in this way. The benefits far outweigh the risks: of every 1,000 people treated with aspirin, there will be fourteen fewer heart attacks and four fewer non-bleeding strokes.

Finally, as with any medication, there are a small number of people who cannot tolerate aspirin. But if you notice what you think is any allergic reaction, consult your doctor immediately.

Who Should Avoid Aspirin?   Obviously, anyone who's truly allergic to aspirin should avoid taking it. And because aspirin is a blood thinner, anyone who suffers from a bleeding disorder, such as hemophilia, should avoid aspirin as well. For the same reason, patients scheduled for some kinds of surgery may be told to avoid aspirin for a few days before the operation and for a period afterward as well—although a recent study suggests that aspirin may be beneficial for bypass-surgery patients. Finally, if you are already taking other blood-thinning medications, you should consult with your doctor before adding aspirin.

These concerns aside, however, the bottom line is that aspirin's benefits far outweigh its risks. It is cheap, readily available, and safe for the vast majority of heart disease sufferers at the dosages recommended by the American Heart Association/American College of Cardiology guidelines. For every ten people who are saved from a heart attack or stroke by aspirin, only one will suffer any major aspirin-related complications.

Frequently Asked Questions

Q: DO OTHER PAIN RELIEVERS PROTECT THE HEART LIKE ASPIRIN DOES?

Among all the commonly used over-the-counter pain relievers—acetaminophen (Tylenol), ibuprofen (Advil, Motrin), naproxen (Aleve, Naprosyn), indomethacin (Indocin)—only aspirin has been proven definitively to protect the heart. Like aspirin, some pain relievers such as ibuprofen, naproxen, and indomethacin also have anti-inflammatory properties and can inhibit platelets (which are important for clotting), though their effect is temporary, while aspirin's is permanent. Although some studies suggest that these other medications may also help to protect the heart, these studies are not definitive. And acetaminophen (Tylenol), for example, is not believed to have any effect on the heart. Because so much research has been done on aspirin, it is the only over-the-counter pain reliever that has the support of cardiology experts. Some experts believe that ibuprofen should not be taken with aspirin, but this position is still controversial. Taking some of the other pain relievers (except Tylenol) with aspirin may increase your risk of stomach irritation; it is not clear that it helps or hurts the protective effects of aspirin. Of note, Vioxx (rofecoxib) was recently withdrawn from the market because of evidence that it increases the risk of heart attacks and strokes.

Q: IS IT BETTER TO TAKE BUFFERED OR COATED ASPIRIN INSTEAD OF PLAIN TABLETS?

No. Drug companies claim that "buffered" or "enteric-coated" aspirin helps protect against stomach irritation, but the research that has been done on these claims is inconclusive—and even contradictory. Indeed, a study that examined all research to date on these forms of aspirin concluded that they do not reduce the risk of stomach or intestinal bleeding. They simply tend to cost more.

Q: WILL A HIGHER-DOSE ASPIRIN TABLET BE MORE EFFECTIVE THAN A LOWER ONE?

Again, no. Research shows that aspirin provides the same heart protection benefit whether you take a low-strength tablet (at least

75 mg) or a higher one. Baby aspirin is usually 81 mg. Some people prefer the 325 mg dose because, ironically, it's often less expensive than tablets with smaller dosage; they simply cut the higher dose tablets in half. However, there is no clear evidence that a lower dose reduces your risk of stomach irritation.

Q: IS GRAPE JUICE A SUBSTITUTE FOR ASPIRIN?

A few studies have suggested that substances called *flavonoids*, contained in purple grape juice, can inhibit platelets from forming clots. Other juices—orange, white grape, grapefruit—can't do this because they are low in this substance. But it hasn't been demonstrated that purple grape juice can decrease the risk of heart disease, so it cannot be used as a substitute for aspirin.

Q: CAN CHOCOLATE SUBSTITUTE FOR ASPIRIN?

Some scientists are actually doing research on the ability of chocolate to inhibit platelets (and clotting) and promote blood flow. Chocolate contains the same flavonoids as grape juice. One study showed that drinking a cocoa drink for four days had a similar, though less strong effect, as taking a baby aspirin. Wouldn't it be fun for doctors to start prescribing chocolate for your heart? Unfortunately, that is not going to happen anytime soon. This research may provide insight into new ways of treating heart disease, but no one is suggesting that any food that contains flavonoids, including chocolate, should substitute for aspirin. By the way, green and black tea also have an abundant amount of flavonoids.

Q: ARE SOME PEOPLE RESISTANT TO THE EFFECT OF ASPIRIN?

Yes. Recent research indicates that for perhaps one in ten people aspirin will not prevent platelets from forming clots. The test that can indicate who will be aspirin-resistant is not yet in wide use, though some researchers want all patients taking aspirin to have this test.

Q: WHAT ABOUT COMBINING ASPIRIN AND IBUPROFEN?

Some researchers have raised concerns that ibuprofen (and perhaps some other drugs like it) may blunt the benefit of aspirin for patients with heart disease. This issue is important because many people are taking both of these medications. For now, it is far from clear whether this concern has any merit. Studies have not consistently supported the concern—but the methods of the different studies make them hard to compare. For now, it seems prudent to combine them only if you really need both (good advice for any medication). This topic is likely to remain controversial for some time.

Clopidogrel (brand name: Plavix) Like aspirin, clopidogrel is a blood thinner that affects the ability of platelets to form clots. If you are unable to take aspirin, research suggests that clopidogrel is at least as effective as aspirin in reducing your risk of a heart attack or stroke. Indeed, one study of more than 10,000 people who suffered from heart disease, stroke, or narrowing of the arteries showed that clopidogrel might work slightly better than aspirin at lowering a patient's risk of suffering another heart attack or stroke, and of dying. Clopidogrel's potential side effects—stomach irritation and bleeding—are the same as aspirin's. Clopidogrel can cause a rash in rare cases and, in even rarer instances (affecting only a few people for every 1,000 treated), can adversely affect white blood cells.

Consequently, the American Heart Association/American College of Cardiology guidelines recommend that anyone with heart disease who is unable to take aspirin take clopidogrel instead. For patients who have just suffered a heart attack, clopidogrel is typically prescribed *in addition to* aspirin for at least nine months (see the section After a Heart Attack, on pages 103–105).

Frequently Asked Questions

Q: IF CLOPIDOGREL IS SO EFFECTIVE, WHY DO DOCTORS RECOMMENDED ASPIRIN FIRST?

While clopidogrel may be slightly more effective than aspirin, it is expensive and requires a prescription; aspirin is cheap and doesn't. Also, although one study has suggested that clopidogrel may be better than aspirin, experts tend to be conservative with the results of just a single study, no matter how impressive those results may be. Consequently, at this point clopidogrel is not recommended first.

Warfarin (brand name: Coumadin)   Warfarin is a potent anticoagulant (blood thinner) commonly prescribed after major surgery and for people who have mechanical heart valve replacements, as well as for patients with atrial fibrillation (also called an "irregular heartbeat") to prevent the formation of dangerous blood clots. The benefit of warfarin is the prevention of stroke—this blood thinner can dramatically reduce your risk of stroke if you have atrial fibrillation. It is particularly important for you to ask your doctor about warfarin if you have atrial fibrillation and are not taking this drug—many people in this country with atrial fibrillation who could benefit from warfarin are not receiving it.

Research has shown that warfarin also can have benefits for patients with heart disease similar to those of aspirin and clopidogrel, and so it has been recommended for patients who can't tolerate those drugs. A study from Norway suggests that it may even be better at reducing the risk of future heart problems. But warfarin is a more powerful blood thinner than the others and, as a result, has a higher risk of causing internal bleeding. It is so powerful that patients taking it must have a regular blood test to keep track of how well it's working. The test, called an International Normalized Ratio (or, INR), measures certain aspects of the clotting process. The best level for you depends on your condition. However, the risk of bleeding increases markedly when the INR level rises above 3.0 seconds, and that's the most common concern with this medication. Minor bleeding can be common—bruising, nosebleeds, cuts when shaving that bleed excessively, among others. These effects occur in one of every six people taking the medication. (Heavier menstrual bleeding is rare.) Major bleeding is less common, though more dangerous when it occurs. The INR level is related to the dose of warfarin taken, but it can also be affected by diet and other medications. That's one reason why it is monitored carefully and regularly.

Frequently Asked Questions

Q: IF WARFARIN IS SUCH A POTENT BLOOD THINNER, WHY ISN'T IT THE PREFERRED DRUG FOR PROTECTING AGAINST HEART DAMAGE?

Warfarin has the same disadvantages as clopidogrel: it costs more than aspirin (though not as much as clopidogrel) and requires a prescription. But it has the additional disadvantage of needing to be monitored frequently through blood tests, which are also costly, and inconvenient as well. Moreover, if not monitored closely it can cause severe bleeding.

★★★Beta-Blockers

Your body is equipped with an extraordinary variety of internal communication systems—chemical and electrical pathways through which signals are communicated. The primitive "fight or flight" response we all feel when suddenly confronted with something stressful is regulated by a system of *beta-adrenergic receptors* that exist in tissues throughout your body. They respond to the release of a hormone produced in your adrenal gland by, among other things, speeding up your heart and increasing its demand for oxygen and preparing you to confront the challenge. That's exactly what you want to have happen when faced with an emergency—unless, that is, you have heart disease. In that case, the very same response system your body has designed to save you can, instead, hurt you.

So-called beta-blockers—invented by Scottish researcher Sir James Black in the 1960s—keep those receptors from responding, keep your heart from racing and beating hard, and thus reduce your heart's need for oxygen. Black created them to reduce the pain of angina, but a 1981 study found that beta-blockers helped prevent second heart attacks. The researchers were so excited by this finding that they ended the study early so that patients in the control group (the ones taking the placebo) could also take beta-blockers. Other studies have since confirmed this result, demonstrating that beta-blockers can reduce the odds of having another heart attack or of dying by at least 25 percent. And that's not all. Beta-blockers have also been found to be effective at preventing and treating irregular heartbeats, heart failure, and high blood pressure, reducing stress on the heart, and decreasing the amount of injury that occurs during a heart attack. Indeed, beta-blockers may even decrease scarring of the heart muscle following a heart attack.

What the Guidelines Say   Since Sir James Black's discovery, for which he received the Nobel Prize, beta-blockers have become the cornerstone medication for people with heart problems, from

Commonly Used Beta-Blockers and Their Brand Names	
Generic Name	**Brand Name**
acebutolol	Sectral
atenolol	Tenormin
betaxolol	Kerlone
bisoprolol	Zebeta
carteolol	Cartrol
carvedilol	Coreg
labetalol	Normodyne
metoprolol	Lopressor
metoprolol extended release	Toprol XL
nadolol	Corgard
penbutolol	Levatol
pindolol	Visken
propanolol	Inderal
propanolol long-acting	Inderal LA
sotalol	Betapace
timolol	Blocadren

angina to heart attacks to heart failure. If you've had any of these conditions, the chances are your doctor will prescribe a beta-blocker for you to take indefinitely. Many kinds of beta-blockers have been created over the years, including acebutolol, atenolol, betaxolol, bisoprolol, carteolol, carvedilol, labetalol, metoprolol, nadolol, penbutolol, pindolol, propanolol, sotalol, and timolol.

Precisely which type and dose of beta-blocker you take will depend upon the heart condition for which your doctor prescribes it and how well you tolerate its side effects. In addition, beta-blockers differ in how long they last in the body. Longer-lasting beta-blockers can be taken less frequently. You'll want to discuss all of these factors with your doctor when considering which beta-blocker to choose.

Common Beta-Blocker Side Effects   Most people taking beta-blockers experience few side effects. When they do, these effects typically are minor and disappear with time. Fatigue is the most common side effect—and, consequently, athletic patients may feel that they are unable to perform at peak levels. Sexual dysfunction has also been associated with beta-blockers. But both of these side effects are not very common. In an analysis of a large number of clinical trials, involving more than 30,000 individuals, the researchers found that beta-blockers were associated with increased fatigue in only 18 of every 1,000 people treated and with sexual dysfunction in only 5 of every 1,000 people. Since these same symptoms can occur in any patient with heart disease, they can often be wrongly attributed to beta-blockers. In addition to these effects, patients with peripheral vascular disease (narrowing of the arteries to the legs) may find that the pain they feel when walking increases. A few patients may find that their heartbeat slows so profoundly that they feel weak or dizzy. In general, however, the risk of these side effects is far offset by the benefit of the medications. Also, some people believe that beta-blockers increase the risk of depression, but the studies have not supported that concern.

Beta-Blocker Risks and Benefits   If you already have a very slow heart rate or if you have a propensity for a slow heart rate and do not have a pacemaker, you shouldn't be taking beta-blockers (this is something to discuss with your doctor). In addition, if you suffer from asthma, you should know that beta-blockers can trigger or worsen asthma symptoms. If your asthma is mild to moderate, though, studies show that some types of beta-blockers may be safe for you.

For the vast majority of people with heart disease, however, the benefits of beta-blockers far outweigh the risks. If you're concerned about possible side effects or risks, you and your doctor may consider a trial period. If you do not tolerate beta-blockers, they can be discontinued.

Frequently Asked Questions

Q: CAN I TAKE A BETA-BLOCKER IF I HAVE CHRONIC OBSTRUCTIVE PULMONARY DISEASE (COPD) OR EMPHYSEMA?

COPD, also known as emphysema or chronic lung disease, is a condition that commonly, but not always, occurs as a result of long-term smoking. It limits your ability to breathe, and patients with this condition often need many medications. Some people with this problem cannot take beta-blockers. Others, with milder forms of lung disease, can give beta-blockers a try. While beta-blockers can affect many organs in the body, including the lungs, certain beta-blockers are "cardioselective," which means that their actions target the heart more specifically. These beta-blockers, such as metoprolol and atenolol, are safer for patients who have COPD.

Q: ARE THERE BETA-BLOCKERS IN EYEDROPS?

Certain types of eyedrops, designed to treat glaucoma, contain beta-blockers. Even though the medication goes in the eyes, it can be absorbed into the body and affect the heart. Sometimes the doctor who is prescribing the eyedrops is different from the doctor prescribing your heart medications, so be sure that all your doctors know about all the medications you are taking. Some people do take beta-blockers by eyedrops and pills at the same time—but only under close supervision and with careful attention to the dosage.

Q: SHOULD I TAKE BETA-BLOCKERS IF I HAVE HEART FAILURE?

Heart failure is a condition in which the pumping or filling function of the heart is impaired. Since beta-blockers relax the heart, doctors have long been concerned that these drugs might further weaken a damaged heart. Now, however, there is strong evidence that the effect is just the opposite and beta-blockers have become a preferred therapy for patients with heart failure. In a patient with heart failure, a beta-blocker must be started at a low dose and then increased slowly, but it produces a remarkable benefit.

Q: DO BETA-BLOCKERS CAUSE DEPRESSION?

Some researchers have suggested that beta-blockers may cause depression. Although they do affect the brain as well as the heart, a comprehensive survey of all the studies of beta-blockers failed to show that people taking beta-blockers suffer from depression any more than people who do not take them. Therefore, expert opinion is that beta-blockers do not put you at a substantially higher risk of being depressed.

★★★ACE Inhibitors

Like beta-blockers, angiotensin-converting enzyme (ACE) inhibitors keep your body from doing something it would normally do—in this case, releasing an enzyme called angiotensin II, which causes your blood pressure to rise. As I explained in Strategy #1, high blood pressure makes your heart work harder. If your heart is already weak, working harder will weaken it further, which can worsen your heart disease and even lead to heart failure.

From Venom to Virtue   In the banana plantations of southwestern Brazil, field workers who were bitten by a pit viper snake called *Bothros jararaca* typically collapsed, due to a sudden and catastrophic drop in their blood pressure. In the late 1960s, scientists discovered why: the snake venom contained a potent substance that inhibited the normal functioning of something called angiotensin-converting enzymes. Scientists reasoned that if inhibiting these enzymes could drop normal blood pressure to below-normal levels, it might also drop high blood pressure to normal levels. That's exactly what the drugs they developed—called "ACE inhibitors"—do, though more safely than the snake venom.

Commonly Used ACE Inhibitors and Their Brand Names	
Generic Name	**Brand Name**
benazepril	Lotensin
captopril	Capoten
enalapril	Vasotec
fosinopril	Monopril
lisinopril	Prinivil or Zestril
moexepril	Univasc
perindopril	Aceon
quinapril	Accupril
ramipril	Altace
trandolapril	Mavik

These drugs have proven to be exceptionally effective, and not just for reducing blood pressure. In the 1990s, large trials of ACE inhibitors showed that they could not only treat high blood pressure but also improve the survival of people with heart failure and of certain patients who had suffered a heart attack. A more recent study suggested that all patients who have had a heart attack may benefit from ACE inhibitors. Among patients with heart disease, many of whom were already also taking aspirin and beta-blockers, ACE inhibitors reduced the risk of heart attack by 20 percent, stroke by 30 percent, and death from heart attack or stroke by 25 percent. Moreover, researchers are beginning to discover that ACE inhibitors can protect people with diabetes from developing kidney disease.

What the Guidelines Say   If you have heart disease, you should take an ACE inhibitor every day for the rest of your life. If you have heart disease or narrowed arteries but have never had a heart attack or heart failure, it may still be a good idea for you to take an ACE inhibitor.

ACE Inhibitor Side Effects   The most common side effect of ACE inhibitors is a dry cough, which affects 5 to 10 percent of people taking the medication. If the cough is too bothersome, your doctor may recommend an alternative medication, called an *angiotensin receptor blocker* (ARB, described below). In addition, some people experience dizziness when they first start taking ACE inhibitors, but this symptom usually decreases with time. Other less common side effects of ACE inhibitors include fatigue, headache, stomach upset, and rashes. If you experience any of these side effects, discuss them with your doctor.

ACE Inhibitor Risks and Benefits   If, in addition to heart disease, you also suffer from severe kidney disease or kidney failure, you'll need to consult with your doctors about using ACE inhibitors since they can occasionally worsen the function of the kidneys. More often, however, ACE inhibitors are used to prevent kidney failure, particularly in people with diabetes. If you have an elevated potassium level, ACE inhibitors can also create an increased risk. And of course, should you prove to be allergic to them, you should not continue taking ACE inhibitors.

Overall, however, the risks and side effects of ACE inhibitors are far offset by their dramatic benefits.

Frequently Asked Questions

Q: WHAT IS THE DIFFERENCE BETWEEN ACE INHIBITORS AND ANGIOTENSIN II RECEPTOR BLOCKERS (ARBS)?

Like ACE inhibitors, ARBs lower high blood pressure and help patients with heart failure. This is why patients who develop side effects from ACE inhibitors, such as a dry cough, are often switched to an ARB. Clinical studies have just recently shown that ARBs, like

ACE inhibitors, can also have a powerful effect on lowering a person's risk for heart attack and stroke if he or she has abnormal heart function. ARBs are considered a "second-line" strategy because more evidence is available to support the use of ACE inhibitors. You should know that the guidelines support the use of ARBs, though less strongly than ACE inhibitors, as ARBs are a relatively newer medication that have been studied less extensively than ACE inhibitors.

Commonly Used ARBs and Their Brand Names	
Generic Name	**Brand Name**
candesartan	Atacand
eprosartan	Tevetan
irbesartan	Avapro
losartan	Cozaar
olmesartan	Benicar
telmisartan	Micardis
valsartan	Diovan

After a Heart Attack

Once you've had a heart attack or other major heart problem needing hospital care, the chance that you will experience other heart problems is high. In such cases, your doctor may combine some of the medications we have discussed in this section to minimize your risk of additional heart problems in the future.

What the Guidelines Say   If you have had a heart attack, the American Heart Association/American College of Cardiology guidelines recommend that you take the following medications:

- aspirin, 75 to 325 mg per day (if you have a medical reason not to take aspirin, you should take clopidogrel, 75 mg daily instead);

- clopidogrel, along with aspirin, every day for nine months, starting the day you leave the hospital if you've had a heart attack that is called a non-ST segment-elevation heart attack (a distinction based on the ECG);

- a beta-blocker (unless you have a medical reason not to);

- a statin, especially if your LDL cholesterol is still over 100 mg/dL;

- an ACE inhibitor; and

- an aldosterone blocker (e.g., spironolactone or eplerenone) for patients with abnormal heart function and symptoms of heart failure (e.g., shortness of breath, swelling of the legs). This therapy should be used with caution if you have kidney problems or a propensity to high potassium levels.

As it turns out, the medications that have been shown to help protect a person who has just had a heart attack from having another one are almost the same as those that have been proven to benefit people with heart disease over the long term.

Post–Heart Attack Medication Combinations

Aspirin and Clopidogrel   One main difference between the guidelines for treating any patient with heart disease and those for treating a patient who has just had a heart attack is the recommendation to take *both* clopidogrel and aspirin for nine months after certain types of heart attacks.

A large clinical study showed that heart attack patients with a certain ECG pattern (a non-ST segment elevation—something you can ask your doctor about) who were given both clopidogrel and aspirin for nine months after they left the hospital had a 20 percent lower risk of having another heart attack, stroke, or dying when compared with patients who took only aspirin during that period. Patients who took the clopidogrel-and-aspirin combination did have a higher risk of bleeding, but the overall benefits of this treatment outweighed the risk.

A new study also shows that taking both clopidogrel and aspirin for one year after undergoing angioplasty or stenting (a procedure done to widen a narrowed coronary artery) lowered the risk of having a heart attack, stroke, or dying by 27 percent without significantly increasing the risk of bleeding. These results have not yet been translated into mainstream practice, but they do serve to highlight the potential importance of using clopidogrel and aspirin together in certain situations.

ASPIRIN AND WARFARIN   An alternative approach for people who have just had a heart attack is the combination of warfarin and aspirin. Recent clinical studies suggest that taking warfarin plus aspirin for a year or more after having a heart attack may reduce your risk of subsequent heart attack or stroke, or of dying, compared with taking aspirin alone. The combination therapy does carry with it an increased risk of bleeding, but the researchers in favor of this combined approach believe that this risk is heavily outweighed by the potential benefit.

The newest studies suggest that the warfarin dose needed to gain this benefit over aspirin is slightly higher than the dose that has been used in the past to treat people with only heart disease. In light of this, and because of the increased risk of bleeding, doctors will probably continue to be cautious about prescribing warfarin. However, warfarin plus aspirin may be a good option for people who have a high risk of forming blood clots.

You should know that it is still unclear if warfarin plus aspirin is better than clopidogrel plus aspirin. More research in this area will help doctors and patients to better understand the role of warfarin in treating people just after a heart attack. In the meantime, clopidogrel may be favored because it does not require the monitoring that is essential when using warfarin. (See Appendix D, "Drug Interactions," for more information about potentially troublesome combinations of medications.)

I remember my heart attack so well. It was devastating. I was fifty-nine years old. I had just returned from my daughter's graduation. I remember it was at night and I began to feel a discomfort in my chest. It felt like three burning spots. At first I thought I had indigestion, so I took an antacid and went to bed. I awoke at midnight with the pain and called my son to take me to the emergency room. He drove so fast. I told him that I was not having a heart attack but would have one if he did not slow down.

At first they treated me for indigestion, but then I was told I was having a heart attack. I could not believe it. I thought that I had done everything "right." I never smoked or drank. My cholesterol was fine. Why was this happening to me? I started crying. It seemed like my whole world was turned upside down. My mother and father had both had heart attacks. I was scared.

That early period was really rough. I used a lot of prayer. I felt depressed and, at first, couldn't do anything. After two weeks the doctor told me that I needed to go to cardiac rehabilitation. I remember driving there and being so weak that I could barely close the door. I took the elevator up and needed to sit down to rest. After a while I started on the treadmill and went very slowly. Bit by bit I could do more and soon I felt like a different person.

I made up my mind that I wanted to live. I had to get over my fear of everything. I did not want another heart attack. I started to exercise regularly and eat right. I lost thirty pounds that first year. The key was smaller portions and few snacks between meals.

The big decision I made was to put myself first—for the first time in my life. I spent my whole life putting others ahead of myself. Now I take care of myself. In the morning, after thirty minutes of prayer, I do thirty minutes on the treadmill. I do it for me.

I pay close attention to my medications. I am on a beta-blocker and a medication to treat my cholesterol. I also take aspirin. I use a pillbox that helps me to remember to take my medications.

My advice to others is that they need to make the decision to put themselves first. Self-esteem is the key. You need to learn to take charge of your life—take responsibility for your health. It has been seven years since my heart attack, and I have never felt better.

—Anna

CHAPTER 3

Beyond the Key Strategies

As we've seen, the seven key strategies described in the preceding chapter are the therapies that panels of experts—principally, but not exclusively, those organized by the American Heart Association/American College of Cardiology—have agreed will work to help you take charge of your heart disease. But the American medical establishment is cautious, and with good reason. What these expert panels recommend in their guidelines influences the treatment decisions of thousands of physicians and the lives of hundreds of thousands of patients around the country. Consequently, their guidelines include only those treatment strategies that research has demonstrated conclusively to be effective.

That doesn't mean these are the only treatment approaches for heart disease, or that other treatments might not be good for your heart. Far from it. Obviously, no treatment that presents more risks than benefits, or that may actually harm you, will make it into the guidelines. But other treatments that seem to hold some promise for helping you control your heart disease may not yet have been incorporated into the guidelines simply because, in the opinion of the experts, research on them is either insufficient or scientifically inconclusive. Indeed, the National Institutes of Health recently created a new agency to investigate treatments outside the mainstream of medicine.

This chapter explores five additional treatment strategies for heart disease. If you and your doctor decide to incorporate any of them into your heart disease recovery program, this chapter will help you understand where the research on them currently stands, where there is controversy, and where there may even, in some instances, be some danger.

★★Managing Your Diet

There's the old saying "You are what you eat," and it's especially true in heart disease. It's not just a matter of Americans having "supersized" themselves into an obesity epidemic, although that is certainly the case. Indeed, researchers have proven that the main reason so many Americans are struggling with their weight is simply because we are eating more and exercising less.

One recent study shows that average food portions in the United States have significantly increased in size over the last few decades. Researchers looked carefully at the average portion sizes from 1977 to 1996 and found a remarkable trend. The average portion size for salty snacks increased by 93 calories. Hamburgers increased by about 100 calories. Soft drinks increased by about 50 calories. These changes may seem modest for any given portion—but over the course of a year they add up.

Quantity isn't the only issue. It's increasingly clear that what you eat is as important as how much you eat—and has a direct effect on both your propensity for heart disease and your ability to recover from it.

If that's the case, you might ask: Why isn't diet management one of the key strategies in the previous section of this book? Simple, really: We don't know enough yet about the best approach to diet. Most of the studies that demonstrate the heart benefits of certain approaches to diet are what scientists call "observational studies." They are called "observational" because they involve observing people over time. In many cases researchers work backward to figure out what factors might have made a difference in whether someone did or did not develop the disease in question. In this case, the studies have tracked the diet-related experiences of large groups of people over time. But in observational studies it is often difficult to disentangle the effects of diet from other factors, many of which may not even be measured. For example, people with healthy diet habits may also exercise more, deal more effectively with stress, and have other health habits that affect their long-term well-being as significantly as their diet. As we've already seen in earlier chapters, we know with certainty that diet is a crucial factor in managing blood pressure, blood sugar, cholesterol, and obesity, but research on the direct effect of dietary choices on heart disease is still emerging.

Much of what we do know about diet and heart disease comes from three long-term observational studies: the Nurses' Health Study (involving more than 86,000 female nurses); the Physicians' Health Study (involving 22,000 male physicians); and the Health Professionals' Follow-Up Study (involving 50,000 male dentists, veterinarians, pharmacists, optometrists, osteopathic physicians, and podiatrists). In each study, participants completed detailed questionnaires about their dietary and lifestyle habits and then had their health tracked for more than a decade. Since none of the participants had heart disease at the outset of these studies, researchers have been able to examine the role of diet in those who subsequently developed heart disease as well as those who did not. As a result of these and other studies, doctors and nutritionists are revising the definition of a healthy diet.

Rebuilding the Pyramid

Remember the "food pyramid" you learned about in school? It was an attempt by nutritionists at the U.S. Department of Agriculture (USDA) to give people a sense of the proper proportions of types of food they should be eating every day. At the base of the pyramid, representing the largest proportion of food that should be in your diet, were the starches—bread, cereal, rice, and pasta, for example. At the peak of the pyramid, representing the smallest quantity recommended, were fats—butter, oils, margarine. In between were all the other food groups—fruits and vegetables, dairy, and proteins. But if you never learned about the food pyramid in school, you needn't worry: it's changed. Research conducted over the past three or four decades has made it clear that some of the blocks in the pyramid were in the wrong place and that some of the items in each block were, in some cases, more complicated than they'd first seemed. A diet high in starches, for example, can lead to obesity and other health problems in a sedentary population. There seems to be a difference in the health effects of whole grains compared with refined grains. Fruits and vegetables have been found to have a variety of disease-preventing properties. And while some fats are clearly bad for you, others are actually beneficial.

As a result of these discoveries, the USDA is working on a revision of the food pyramid. Meanwhile, some experts have proposed that whole-grain foods and plant oils (e.g., olive, canola, soy, corn, sunflower, and peanut) form the foundation of the new pyramid. The next level up would be vegetables and fruit, followed by nuts and legumes. Fish, poultry, and eggs would be next. At the top, representing the smallest quantity of the diet, would be red meat, butter, and refined carbohydrates. Alcohol, which we explore in the next chapter, is also recommended in moderation. Although this new pyramid has not yet been widely accepted, it is based upon stronger evidence than the old pyramid.

The American Heart Association has modified its dietary guidelines as well. We'll look at the research on several of the major food groups in a moment, but here's a summary of what the AHA recommends to keep your heart healthy:

- Eat a variety of fruits and vegetables and choose at least 5 servings per day.

- Eat a variety of grain products, including whole grains, and choose at least 6 servings per day.

- Include fat-free and low-fat milk products, fish, legumes (beans), skinless poultry, and lean meats.

- Choose fats and oils with 2 grams or less of saturated fat per tablespoon, such as liquid and tub margarines, canola oil, and olive oil.

- Choose foods that are low in saturated fat, trans fat, and cholesterol.

- Limit your intake of foods that are high in calories and low in nutrition, such as sugary soft drinks and candy.

- Eat less than 6 grams of salt (sodium chloride) per day (2.4 grams of sodium).

Most packaged foods now carry nutrition labels that let you know how much of certain items—calories, various fats, carbohydrates, proteins, vitamins, and minerals, for example—is contained in a standardized serving. But other aspects of food labeling, like sodium content, can be confusing. Here's a key to what the advertising really means in the case of salt (by way of reference, there are 2.6 grams of sodium in a single teaspoon of table salt, and there are 1,000 milligrams in a gram):

Salt Content on Food Labels	
What it says:	**What it means:**
"Sodium-free"	less than 5 mg of sodium per serving
"Very low-sodium"	35 mg or less per serving
"Low-sodium"	140 mg or less per serving
"Unsalted"	no salt added, but it still contains the sodium that is a natural part of the food itself
Adapted from the American Heart Association, 2002, and from Facts about the DASH Diet, National Institutes of Health, National Heart, Lung, and Blood Institute, Bethesda, 1998.	

Good and Bad Fats

As researchers have begun to understand the effects of different kinds of fats on both "good" and "bad" cholesterol in your bloodstream, they've established new guidelines for "good" and "bad" fats in your diet. Bad fats include saturated fats, trans fatty acids (trans fats), and cholesterol. Saturated fats are found in whole milk, cream, ice cream, whole-milk cheeses, butter, lard, and meats. They're also found in palm, palm kernal, and coconut oils and in coconut butter.

Fat Content on Food Labels	
What it says:	What it means:
"Fat-free"	less than 0.5 g of fat per serving
"Low-saturated fat"	1 g or less per serving
"Low fat"	3 g or less per serving
"Reduced fat"	at least 25 percent less fat than the regular version
"Lean"	less than 10 g of fat, less than 4 g of saturated fat, and less than 95 mg of cholesterol
"Extra lean"	less than 5 g of fat, less than 2 g of saturated fat, and less than 95 mg of cholesterol
"Light (lite)"	at least a third fewer calories or no more than half the fat of the regular product or no more than half the sodium of the regular product
Adapted from the American Heart Association, 2002, and from Facts about the DASH Diet, National Institutes of Health, National Heart, Lung, and Blood Institute, Bethesda, 1998.	

Trans fats are made when food manufacturers add hydrogen to vegetable oil. They are found in the partially hydrogenated vegetable oils used to make hard "stick" margarine (but not soft "tub" margarine) and are also typically used in commercially manufactured cookies, cakes, crackers, french fries, fried onions, and doughnuts, among other snack foods. In the past, scientists have focused on the dangers of saturated fats, but new research by the Institute of Medicine suggests that trans fats increase bad (LDL) cholesterol and also decrease good (HDL) cholesterol. No other dietary factor has both of these bad effects, and trans fats can damage arteries as much as or more than saturated fats.

Cholesterol exists on its own, of course, in varying concentrations in most animal products—meats (and especially organ meats, like liver or heart), egg yolks, dairy products, and, to a much lesser extent, fish and poultry.

On the other hand, it is increasingly clear that some fats actually help lower your bad cholesterol levels and increase good cholesterol. These good fats include polyunsaturated fats such as safflower, sesame, soy, corn, and sunflower oils, seeds and nuts, and monounsaturated fats such as olive, canola and peanut oils, and avocados.

Cutting Saturated Fat When You Cook	
Saturated Fat, Measured in Grams Per Tablespoon **(1 g = 1,000 mg)**	
HIGH SATURATED FAT	
butter	7.0 to 8.0 g
lard	5.0 g
margarine blend (60% corn oil & 40% butter)	4.0 g
chicken fat	3.8 g
wheat germ oil	2.6 g
peanut salad or cooking oil	2.3 g
LOW SATURATED FAT	
soft or corn margarine (hydrogenated & regular)	2.0 g
soybean salad or cooking oil (hydrogenated)	2.0 g
sesame salad or cooking oil	1.9 g
olive salad or cooking oil	1.8 g
corn salad or cooking oil	1.7 g
almond oil	1.1 g
canola oil	1.0 g

Adapted from the American Heart Association, 2002, and from Facts about the DASH Diet, National Institutes of Health, National Heart, Lung, and Blood Institute. Bethesda, 1998.

On the basis of these new findings, researchers and physicians encourage you to use polyunsaturated and monounsaturated fats wherever possible. It's worth noting, however, that even these "good" fats are high in calories and therefore should be consumed in moderation.

★★Fish and Your Heart

Some years ago, researchers discovered that members of the Inuit tribe, native to the Arctic, had a much lower rate of heart disease than non-natives. In time, the researchers concluded that the reason was that the Inuit diet consists mainly of fish that are high in certain types of fats. These fish contain what scientists call "long-chain n-3 fatty acids" (including omega-3 and omega-6 fatty acids) that are polyunsaturated and improve cholesterol levels and reduce triglyceride levels in the bloodstream. These fatty acids may reduce the risk of fatal heart rhythms and may have beneficial effects on triglyceride levels and blood clotting.

Subsequently, the Physicians' Health Study found that high blood levels of n-3 fatty acids were related to a greatly lowered risk of sudden death from heart problems. In the Nurses' Health Study researchers found that the more frequently a woman eats fish, the lower her risk of getting heart disease or having a heart attack. The Health Professionals' Study revealed that eating fish at least once per month was associated with an over 40 percent lower risk of stroke.

In addition, there's now evidence that eating fatty fish also helps protect the hearts of people who already have heart disease. One study of more than 11,000 people with heart disease found that taking a 1-gram daily supplement of n-3 polyunsaturated fatty acids (equivalent to 3.5 ounces of salmon or 7 ounces of tuna) lowered their risk of having a fatal heart problem by up to 30 percent. In another study, British heart patients who were advised to eat two servings of oily fish a week for two years had a 29 percent lower risk of death. These studies suggest that eating fatty fish helps heart disease patients.

By the way, the fish themselves do not produce these substances.

The oils are made by small marine organisms that the fish eat. They occur in varying proportions in different fish. In general, the fish that seem to have more oil have more of these fatty acids. High concentrations are found in tuna, sardines, salmon, mackerel, and herring. But it's likely that not all fatty fish are alike in providing these benefits. Mackerel, for example, is a fatty fish that can provide as much as 1 gram of omega-3 fatty acid with each serving. But it also contains nearly 2 grams of saturated fat. Tuna, on the other hand, has between 0.2 and 1.2 grams of omega-3 fatty acid per serving (depending on the type of tuna), but no saturated fat. So it pays to know which fish offer the greatest benefits. How the fish is prepared also matters. Fried, processed, salted, or pickled fish typically contain ingredients, including saturated fats and high concentrations of salt, that pose a risk to heart health that outweighs any possible benefit. As you may remember from earlier sections, regularly consuming food that is high in saturated fats or high in salt can raise your cholesterol or your blood pressure, respectively. So when eating fish, it is best to choose nonfried fish that was not processed or prepackaged.

Given these new findings, the American Heart Association now recommends that everyone eat a full serving of fish two to three times per week. In addition, the AHA recommends that people with heart disease consume approximately 1 gram of fish-derived omega-3 fatty acids, preferably by eating fish itself, though fish-oil supplements (also called "EPA + DHA" capsules) also may be used. What's more, if you have a high triglyceride level in your bloodstream, the AHA recommends that you consume 2 to 4 grams of fish-derived omega-3 fatty acids in the form of EPA + DHA capsules under the supervision of your doctor.

If you take capsules, you should know that they can be taken any time—with meals or not. When they dissolve in the stomach and release the oil, some people have a fishy burp. Some experts suggest that freezing the pills can eliminate this problem. Another solution is taking them at bedtime. Fish-oil capsules vary markedly in price, so you should shop around. And it is best to choose a supplement with an EPA/DHA ratio between 2:1 and 1:2.

Some people are concerned about mercury and other pollutants in fish. It is true that the FDA has issued an advisory that is directed at reducing mercury exposure for women who may become pregnant, pregnant women, nursing mothers, and young children. The advisory states that these groups should avoid shark, swordfish, king mackerel, or tilefish because they contain high levels of mercury. It also expresses a concern about albacore tuna, suggesting that the above groups eat no more than one serving a week. The advisory acknowledges that there are many benefits to eating fish and that it is an important component of a balanced diet. For patients with heart disease, the benefits of eating fish likely far outweigh any concern about mercury or other pollutants. Also, fish-oil capsules do not contain any mercury.

Some people also wonder whether it is better to eat salmon from the wild or from fish farms. Both types of fish are good sources of these fatty acids. A recent report raised some concerns about contaminants in fish from farms. The amount is very small and the benefits of eating the fish seems to far outweigh any concerns.

★★The Importance of Fruits and Vegetables

It's long been known that fruits and vegetables contain substances that help protect against a number of medical conditions, including cancers of the lung, mouth, esophagus, and colon. They may also help prevent breast and prostate cancers. New research suggests that the fiber, minerals, and antioxidants in fruits and vegetables also protect your heart.

A large study that included participants from both the Nurses' Health Study and the Health Professionals' Follow-Up Study found that each extra serving of fruits and vegetables consumed per day was related to a 4 percent lower risk of heart attack and a 6 percent lower risk of stroke. These findings have not been confirmed in a formal clinical trial, and it is possible that the people in this and similar studies who ate more fruits and vegetables were healthier at the outset. But the researchers involved in this study have concluded that increasing your intake of fruits and vegetables could lower your risk of heart problems by 5 to 20 percent over the long term.

★Fiber and Your Heart

Dietary fiber provides many benefits. Certainly it is beneficial for digestive diseases, as studies show it prevents constipation, hemorrhoids, and diverticulosis. Others studies have even suggested that fiber can reduce the risk of certain types of cancer. There is also evidence that fiber is useful as a strategy to reduce the risk of heart disease. A recent study evaluated ten well-conducted studies, including more than 300,000 people. The study showed that fiber from cereals and fruit is associated with a 10 to 30 percent lower risk of heart disease for each 10-grams-per-day increase of total fiber from these sources.

Interestingly, vegetable fiber did not have a strong effect, leading some people to speculate that any beneficial effect of vegetable fiber could be offset by adverse effects of common starchy and highly processed vegetables. Unfortunately the studies often lacked the details needed to understand whether there are differences among the types of vegetables.

Another issue concerns soluble versus insoluble fiber. Both soluble and insoluble fiber pass through our bodies without being digested. Neither of these food components is absorbed into the bloodstream or used as an energy source. Soluble fiber becomes a gel or liquid as it mixes with fluid, and insoluble fiber does not. Many foods contain both soluble and insoluble fiber. The study mentioned above found benefits associated with both types of fiber, though the benefits from soluble fiber were a bit stronger. Nevertheless, the authors stated that their results supported recommendations to increase consumption of *all* types of fiber-rich foods.

★The Benefits of Whole Grains

The grain that's used for most of the starchy foods we eat—white bread, pastries, cakes, cookies, pasta, and white rice, for example—has been "refined." By "refined" we mean that the outer layer of bran and the inner germ of the grain have been removed to make the product whiter. Whole grains, on the other hand, retain those components of the natural grain. That's important, because the bran and germ of grains include fiber, essential fatty acids, and substances called *phytochemicals*, which have been proven to be good for your health. The manufacturers of refined grains and flours often add vitamins and minerals to try to make up for what has been removed, but the resulting products still don't match the health benefits of whole grains. Grain fiber is especially good at reducing cholesterol, and while fiber also exists in some fruits and vegetables, research suggests that grain fiber may be more effective at protecting your heart.

How effective? In the Nurses' Health Study we mentioned earlier, researchers found that women who ate an average of at least three servings of whole grains per day had a 20 percent lower risk of getting heart disease than women who ate little or no whole grains. But we need to be somewhat cautious about these results. In the absence of additional research, it is hard to determine whether these benefits are due to the nutrients and fiber found in whole grains, or to the fact that people who eat whole-grain foods tend to eat and live healthier than other people to begin with. This reservation aside, however, the additional health benefits of eating whole grains (such as improved digestion) suggest that it is a good idea to increase the role of whole grains in your diet.

★The Protective Value of Nuts

As with whole grains, eating nuts seems to have the effect of protecting the heart. The Nurses' Health Study found that women who ate at least five servings of nuts or peanut butter per week had a 20 percent lower rate of developing diabetes. In an earlier study of the same population, researchers also found that women who ate at least five ounces of nuts per week had a 30 percent lower risk of having a heart attack than women who did not eat as many nuts or who ate none at all. In addition, the Physicians' Health Study found that men who ate nuts at least twice a week had a 30 percent lower risk of dying from heart disease than those who never or rarely ate nuts. A few other studies have yielded similar findings, suggesting that nuts contain substances that protect the heart and blood vessels. Still (as with whole grains), more research is needed to determine whether these health effects can be attributed to eating nuts or to the generally healthier diet and lifestyle of those who eat nuts regularly. One promising small study recently showed that when people with high cholesterol snacked on almonds, their LDL cholesterol was lowered by almost 10 percent.

The FDA is actually allowing product labels for walnuts to claim that they lower the risk of heart disease. The label states specifically that "Supportive but not conclusive research shows that eating 1.5 ounces of walnuts per day, as part of a low saturated fat and low cholesterol diet, and not resulting in increased caloric intake, may reduce the risk of coronary heart disease." Other nut producers are petitioning for similar claims. But there is yet another issue to consider: most nuts are very high in calories—a potential problem for people who are trying to lose weight. Therefore, researchers suggest that if you want to increase your consumption of nuts, you must decrease your consumption of refined-grain products or meats, so as to maintain a healthy intake of calories.

Redesigning Your Whole Diet

Keeping track of every one of the specific components of a heart-healthy diet can be complicated and difficult. To make things easier, experts recommend that you simply revise your *entire* diet so that your diet, in effect, keeps track of the right things for you. Their recommendation is that if you have heart disease you should:

- consume foods that are high in unsaturated fats, especially polyunsaturated fats, instead of foods that are high in saturated fats;

- increase your consumption of omega-3 fatty acids found in certain types of fish and plant foods; and

- eat more fruits, vegetables, nuts, and whole grains—and fewer refined grains.

What would a diet based on these principles look like? Well, it certainly wouldn't look like the conventional "Western" diet, which is heavy on red and processed meats, saturated fats, sweets, potatoes, and refined grains. What it would look like is the diet eaten by millions of people in the countries ringing the Mediterranean Sea.

Some years ago, when scientists looked around the world for places where heart disease was uncommon they made a surprising discovery. Heart disease was exceptionally rare among the people of Crete, the largest of the Greek islands. What was surprising about this discovery—coming, as it did, when experts were promoting low-fat diets—was the fact that almost half of all the calories consumed by the people of Crete came from fat! The difference, it soon became clear, was that they were consuming olive oil, which is a primary source of monounsaturated fat—the kind of fat that lowers bad cholesterol and raises good cholesterol. But that's not all. A closer look at what the people on Crete were eating revealed that it was an almost perfect model of what researchers now know is a heart-healthy diet. In fact, it is a model that forms the basis of the cuisines of many Mediterranean countries—Italy, Greece, France, Spain, Portugal, Morocco, Tunisia, Turkey, and Syria, among others.

Though it varies slightly from country to country, this "Mediterranean diet" has a number of common characteristics: It emphasizes:

- an abundance of plant food (fruit, vegetables, breads and cereals, beans, nuts, seeds);

- minimally processed, seasonally fresh, and locally grown foods;

- fresh fruit as the typical daily dessert—while sweets containing concentrated sugars or honey are consumed only a few times per week;

- olive oil as the main source of fat;

- dairy products—mainly cheese and yogurt—eaten in low to moderate amounts;

- up to 4 eggs per week;

- low amounts of red meat; and

- low to moderate amounts of wine, normally with meals (see the following section on alcohol).

Studies suggest that switching to a Mediterranean diet even after already having had a heart attack may lower your risk of having more heart problems, including another heart attack, by as much as 70 percent. So instead of trying to keep track of everything you eat in order to keep your heart healthy, there's an easy and attractive alternative: eat like a Mediterranean!

Frequently Asked Questions

Q: WILL EATING SOY-BASED FOODS HELP MY HEART?

Probably. A number of studies have found that eating soy-based foods can lower LDL (bad) cholesterol and triglycerides while raising HDL (good) cholesterol, and that this effect is strongest in people with the highest cholesterol levels. According to this research, eating approximately 50 grams of soy per day may lower your LDL cholesterol alone by up to 20 mg/dL, or 13 percent. Therefore, the American Heart Association encourages people with very high cholesterol to eat more soy foods in addition to using other cholesterol-lowering therapies. Since it is thought that the effective amount of soy needed to achieve any significant cholesterol benefit is 20 to 50 grams of soy per day, the FDA has allowed food packaging to advertise "heart-healthy" contents if they contain at least 6.25 grams of soy per serving—based on the idea that four servings of that food would be within the effective range. You can also find 6.25 grams of soy protein in many soy-based foods, including: 1 glass of soy milk, 2 to 4 ounces of tofu, or a half an ounce of soy flour.

Q: WHAT ABOUT DRINKING BLACK TEA?

A number of studies suggest that people who drink one or two cups of black tea per day may be at lower risk for developing heart disease and having a heart attack than those who don't. Some experts theorize that the *flavonoids* in black tea prevent plaque buildup and keep blood vessel walls relaxed and healthy. More studies are needed to determine whether black tea on its own truly has a protective effect on the heart. Since drinking this much black tea per day is safe for most people, it is certainly something you can try if it suits your taste. The studies to date suggest that coffee, caffeinated or decaffeinated, probably does not protect the heart. Although green tea contains many of the same substances found in black tea, little is known at this point about the potential heart-protective effects of green tea or other types of teas, including various herbal teas.

Q: CAN GARLIC HELP MY HEART?

It's not clear. A comprehensive analysis of all the trials studying the effects of garlic on cholesterol showed that while it may have some modest ability to lower total cholesterol levels, there are not yet enough data to make a strong recommendation. A review of randomized trials found that garlic reduced total cholesterol levels by 4 to 6 percent. For now, if you have heart disease, you should use more proven approaches for lowering your cholesterol levels. On the other hand, garlic certainly won't hurt you—and it may help.

Q: IS EATING SMALLER, MORE FREQUENT MEALS BETTER FOR MY HEART?

Possibly. A few studies have suggested that eating smaller, more frequent meals may lower your cholesterol. One study surveying over 14,000 people found that those who ate more than six times a day had cholesterol levels that were 5 to 6 mg/dL lower when compared with people who ate only once or twice a day. However, more research is still needed to determine whether increasing the number of mealtimes per day can truly be used as a way to lower cholesterol levels. One danger of eating more frequent meals, of course, is that you may well consume more calories than before, which would be counterproductive. For this reason, and because more needs to be known, it's wise to stick with more conventional methods for lowering your cholesterol for now.

Q: ARE FAT SUBSTITUTES HEALTHIER THAN FATS?

Probably not. When consumers began to be concerned about the amount of fat in their foods, some food companies created fat substitutes, such as olestra, to replace the saturated fats typically used, notably in snack foods such as potato chips. But the real issue here is lowering your overall calorie consumption, not necessarily just lowering fats; "fat free" snacks have calories, too. What's more, fat substitutes such as olestra can decrease the absorption of important dietary nutrients and can have unpleasant side effects for many people. The fact is that the long-term safety of fat substitutes is unknown. Therefore, dietary experts at the American Heart Association recommend that people who choose to consume fat substitutes do so while paying very close attention to their diet overall.

Q: WHAT ABOUT CALORIE RESTRICTION?

Many people believe that the way to longer life is a very restrictive low-calorie diet. Advocates of this approach believe that they can postpone normal aging and avoid the onset of cancer, heart disease, kidney failure, and Alzheimer's disease. There is some scattered evidence that calorie restriction can extend life, but we are far from a scientific consensus on this issue. This evidence comes from animal studies and some observations of the experience of populations that have experienced food deprivation. Thus, the relevance to an average person is not clear. Reducing your food intake to take off extra weight is a good idea. Restricting yourself to a very low-calorie diet is not yet a widely recommended practice. Even if it were, it is doubtful that many people would be able to adhere to it. Several studies are being conducted to determine if this strategy really works.

★Consuming Alcohol

Thirty years ago, scientists studying the incidence of heart disease in different countries around the world found themselves baffled by one particular finding: the French, despite having a diet rich in the kind of fats that cause atherosclerosis, had much lower levels of heart disease than the English. After years of research into what became known as the "French paradox," some scientists think they've solved the puzzle: the French drink a lot of wine. Several large-scale studies have demonstrated that people who regularly have one to three alcoholic drinks a day have a 10 to 40 percent lower risk of developing heart disease than people who don't drink at all. Moderate alcohol consumption also may lower the risk for heart failure and stroke (although drinking large amounts of alcohol may increase that risk).

How Alcohol Protects the Heart

Scientists are not yet certain about how alcohol consumption protects the heart, but there are several possible answers. There are antioxidants in wine, and antioxidants are known to help keep LDL (bad) cholesterol from accumulating into plaques and keep platelets in the blood from forming clots. And a recent review of forty-two studies suggests that alcohol may protect the heart by raising HDL (good) cholesterol levels and lowering levels of fibrinogen, another substance that promotes clotting. There is also evidence that alcohol may fight inflammation in the blood vessels.

Unfortunately, none of the research conducted to date addresses the question of whether drinking alcohol holds benefits for people who already have been diagnosed with heart disease. All we can say with any certainty is that if you have heart disease and have been drinking moderately for some time, it probably isn't hurting you and may well be helping.

What Kind? How Often? How Much?

Early research suggested that wine—and red wine in particular— was more protective against heart disease and cancer than other alcoholic beverages. But a recent study of more than 38,000 men found that when it comes to lowering the risk of heart attack, the type of alcohol (beer, red wine, white wine, or liquor) does not matter. Indeed, this same study concluded that how often you drink alcohol may matter more than what you drink or how much. It turns out that men who drank moderately three to seven days a week were far less likely to develop heart disease than those who drank only one or two days a week.

These research results are not a green light for heavy drinking. The American Heart Association recommends that women consume no more than one alcoholic drink per day and men no more than two. The experts agree that more than three drinks per day is hazardous for anyone—and for many people, problems can develop at even lower levels. Alcohol can be addictive and can lead to physical abuse, accidents, high blood pressure, liver disease, and cancers of the mouth, throat, esophagus, and breast. One recent study showed that as many as half of all moderate drinkers have binge-drinking episodes, which are highly associated with alcohol-impaired driving.

By the way, if you're a non-drinker now, you probably shouldn't start. One study of non-drinkers who took up moderate drinking at midlife concluded that the reduction of heart attack risk was minimal.

Finally, some people should avoid drinking altogether. The American Heart Association has concluded that if you have any of the following conditions, the risks of drinking alcohol far outweigh the benefits:

- a personal or strong family history of alcoholism;

- uncontrolled high blood pressure;

- high blood triglyceride levels;

- heart failure;

- pregnancy;

- porphyria (a genetic disorder);

- pancreatitis (disease of the pancreas); or

- use of medications that interact with alcohol (see Appendix D, "Drug Interactions").

⑦Taking Vitamins and Other Supplements

Since 1994, sales of vitamins and other dietary supplements have soared by well over 50 percent and are estimated to have topped $17 billion annually. One recent study found that up to 70 percent of Americans use vitamins, herbs, and other supplements. What's curious about this is that there is very little evidence that such supplements have any effect on heart disease.

Vitamin E is a good example. Available in vegetables, oils, and nuts, vitamin E is a valuable source of antioxidants. But while magazines, newspapers, and even some doctors have touted vitamin E as "extra insurance" against heart disease, studies involving more than 60,000 people have failed to demonstrate that vitamin E has any effect on the heart at all. What's more, taken in high enough doses, vitamin E may adversely affect heart disease patients who are taking warfarin (brand name: Coumadin) as a blood thinner. (Taking warfarin at the same time as taking vitamin E in doses up to 400 units per day appears to be safe.)

Folic acid (folate) and vitamin B supplements have also been promoted as being good for your heart. There is an amino acid in your blood called *homocysteine* that, at high enough levels, has been associated with an increased risk of heart disease and stroke. Folic acid and, to some extent, vitamins B_{12} and B_6 can lower homocysteine levels in your bloodstream. But it hasn't yet been proven that lowering homocysteine levels has any value for protecting your heart. Early studies suggested that taking folic acid and B vitamins after undergoing angioplasty (a procedure done to open up blocked arteries) helped keep those arteries from closing off again, but clinical trials have failed to show any specific heart-protecting benefits from either folic acid or vitamin B supplements. Moreover, since enriched-grain products are fortified with folic acid, and vitamins B_{12} and B_6 are readily available in meats, dairy products, beans, and grains, anyone following a balanced diet will have little need for supplements.

Some studies have suggested that taking a multivitamin daily may reduce the risk of heart disease and stroke, but this effect may be caused by people who take multivitamins tending to lead healthier lifestyles at the outset. Or it may be that multivitamins benefit heart health only in people who have nutritional deficiencies. Up to this point, there has been no compelling evidence in favor of taking multivitamins for your heart, so if you're following a balanced diet, you most likely don't need them.

Finally, a number of herbal remedies have been promoted to help treat hypertension, lower cholesterol, or protect against heart disease. These include coenzyme Q (ubiquinone), danshen, dong quai, garlic, ginger, ginkgo, ginseng, hellebore, and hawthorn (*crataegus* species). New clinical studies are under way to examine these claims, but as yet there are no reliable research data to demonstrate that any of these alternative medicines have any significant effect on the heart—good or bad.

What do the guidelines say? The U.S. Preventive Services Task Force, an expert group funded by the government, recently conducted a comprehensive review of the medical literature relating to the use of vitamin supplements for cancer and cardiovascular disease prevention. They concluded that the evidence is insufficient to recommend for or against the use of vitamins A, C, or E, multivitamins with folic acid, or antioxidant combinations for the prevention of heart disease (or cancer). They specifically recommended against supplements containing beta carotene. A recent review concluded that vitamin E has no effect.

★Reducing Stress

It would seem a matter of common sense that high levels of stress would tax the heart and, therefore, that stress-reduction techniques would help the heart. But it's not that simple. For example, for some years it was suggested that highly driven, so-called Type A people were more at risk for heart problems than other, more relaxed people. But the truth is that the evidence for this theory is not at all clear. For one thing, researchers found that Type A people were also more likely to be smokers and to have high cholesterol and blood pressure, so lifestyle and diet choices may have been contributing factors no less important than stress. In the end, there simply has not yet been any clear evidence to support the idea that people with Type A behavior are more likely than other people to have heart problems.

On the other hand, there is some scientific evidence to suggest that certain kinds of stress may affect the heart. It does appear that short, acute periods of very high stress can trigger heart problems. For example, researchers found that around the time of the 1994 Northridge, California, earthquake, the rate of sudden cardiac death in that region jumped to over five times the normal rate.

We know less about the effects of longer-term, chronic stress. But a recent review of the small number of studies on stress and heart disease done to date suggests that the following types of everyday stress may possibly be related to heart disease:

- stress that causes depression or anxiety symptoms;

- stress related to work or occupation; and

- stress related to having unstable or too few social relationships.

How, and to what extent, these stresses affect the heart is still unclear. What we do know is that any of these stresses can increase behaviors that are known to be harmful to the heart, such as smoking, eating unhealthy foods, and not exercising. Therefore, taking steps to lower stress in your life may make it easier for you to avoid these behaviors—and give you peace of mind as well.

What kind of stress reduction will protect your heart? The evidence is mixed. One small study showed that relaxation therapy had no effect on lowering blood pressure in individuals with mild hypertension. Yet another small study of twenty-three people in Italy showed that saying the rosary and repeating yoga mantras caused participants to feel more relaxed, slowed their breathing, and improved their heart rate. There is also some evidence to suggest that people with heart disease can lower their risk of future heart problems through formal stress-management training. One technique, developed by a cardiologist, is called the "relaxation response" and is thought to help people manage stress and lower their risk of heart problems. It is thought that incorporating quiet periods of meditation, such as the relaxation response technique, into a person's daily or weekly routine may help to lower blood pressure and other heart problems. But many more studies will be needed before we can say any of these stress-reduction techniques have a true and long-standing effect on heart health. The same is true of antianxiety medications; there simply is no reliable research to suggest that they have significant benefits for reducing the risk of heart disease.

①Using Hormone Therapy

For women experiencing, or who have experienced, menopause, few areas of medical research have seemed more confusing or frustrating than studies on the benefits and risks of hormone replacement therapy. The normal decrease in levels of the hormones estrogen and progesterone, which typically occurs between the ages of 45 and 55, triggers an array of unpleasant symptoms, such as hot flashes and mood swings, and has also long been known to put women at higher risk for osteoporosis and related bone injuries. Research studies have demonstrated that medication that acts like estrogen and progesterone (or, in some instances, only estrogen) can lessen menopause-related symptoms, and protect women against colorectal cancer, osteoporosis, and fractures as well.

Because low estrogen levels in women are also known to be associated with a higher risk for heart disease, researchers thought hormone therapy would also reduce that risk in postmenopausal women, and indeed early studies seemed to confirm that conclusion. Estrogen therapy can raise HDL (good) cholesterol levels by 7 to 8 percent and lower LDL (bad) cholesterol levels in the blood by as much as 10 to 14 percent. In addition, estrogen may also lower other undesirable cholesterol substances in the blood and improve the health of blood vessels in general. On the other hand, estrogen has been shown to increase triglyceride levels as well as levels of certain blood-clotting factors. And while studies revealed that women had a 50 percent higher risk for heart problems and stroke immediately after beginning estrogen therapy, the risk appeared to lessen as time went on, and as a result women were encouraged to continue taking it. Progesterone is typically prescribed along with estrogen because it protects against certain risks caused by using estrogen alone, including endometrial and ovarian cancer, but we know less about how progesterone may affect the heart than we do about estrogen's effects.

A number of studies have sought to understand the benefits and risks of hormone therapy for women, but two merit special mention in the context of heart disease. The Heart and Estrogen/Progestin Replacement Study was a long-term examination of how hormone replacement affects women diagnosed with heart disease. This study found that, when taken by women with heart disease, hormone therapy had no significant long-term benefit and carried significant risks, including a 48 percent increase in gallbladder disease requiring surgery and a doubling of the rate of blood clotting in the legs and lungs.

The results of a more recent study were more dramatic. The Women's Health Initiative Study, sponsored by the National Institutes of Health, was to be a fifteen-year-long study of ways to prevent heart disease, cancer, and osteoporosis in postmenopausal women. When the researchers involved in this study began examining the preliminary results, their findings were so strong and conclusive that they terminated the study of combination therapy early, so as not to prolong the risks to which it exposed the participants. The study discovered that, rather than reducing heart disease risk, combination hormone-replacement therapy caused a 29 percent increase in heart attacks, a 41 percent increase in strokes, doubled the rates of blood clots in the legs and lungs, and increased the risk of breast cancer by 26 percent. In short, not only does combination hormone therapy not protect women with heart disease from further heart problems, it also puts women who do not have heart disease at greater risk of having a heart attack. The study also found that hormone therapy had little effect on a postmenopausal woman's quality of life. The study did reveal some significant benefits of hormone therapy, however, including a 37 percent decline in the risk of colorectal cancer, a 34 percent reduction in hip fractures, and a 24 percent reduction in total fractures due to osteoporosis.

Then, in what some people consider to be the knockout punch for hormone therapy, the study of estrogen alone was also stopped early. After an average of seven years of follow-up, the estrogen therapy did not prevent heart disease and may have increased the risk of stroke.

Even before the release of these new findings, the American Heart Association had announced that hormone therapy for women should not be used as protection against heart disease. The new research underscores this conclusion.

Should all women cease taking hormone medications? Not necessarily. Many women, especially those with a low risk for breast cancer or blood clots, can take these medications in the short term to counteract the most severe symptoms of menopause, including hot flashes, sleep problems, and mood swings. Women who have a high risk of osteoporosis and its related injuries and who have found other treatments for these conditions ineffective may choose to continue with long-term hormone therapy for its proven benefits in this regard. One recent study suggests that women taking these medications for this reason may obtain some protection against heart problems by taking a statin medication at the same time. But the research is clear that you should not take hormone therapy solely to protect against heart disease after menopause. Many postmenopausal women who are at risk of heart disease would be much better advised to use safer, more proven medications, including aspirin and beta-blockers.

Frequently Asked Questions

Q: WHAT ABOUT THE ORNISH PROGRAM?

You may have heard about the program that is promoted by Dr. Dean Ornish. The Ornish Program consists of a plant-based diet with no more than 10 percent of calories from fat, 180 minutes a week of moderate exercise, an hour daily of meditation and other stress-management practices, and biweekly, professionally supervised support group sessions. The approach is low-tech but requires a major commitment. Ornish has demonstrated through imaging studies that this approach has promise. There are no long-term studies of health outcomes, and so it is not yet strongly recommended. A big challenge with this approach is whether people will find the time to make this dramatic change in their life. This program is currently being evaluated by Medicare in 1,800 patients. Preliminary finds are said to be promising.

A PATIENT'S VIEW:

FIGHTING DENIAL

My heart problems date back to the early '90s. I was a forty-eight-year-old professor, and my health was generally good—though I didn't spend much time thinking about it. One day I felt a nagging chest pain when I exerted myself. Soon I couldn't walk a city block. Instead of seeking medical attention I just hoped that it would go away. I guess I just could not escape the power of denial.

I finally did end up seeing a doctor for another problem. When I mentioned the chest pain I was immediately sent for a stress test and then an angiogram. I had three blockages that needed to be opened. Once that was done I thought I had been cured. I didn't hear much about prevention and I didn't really make any changes in my life. In fact I actually gained about twenty pounds and didn't exercise much. I was really out of shape.

Several years later, it happened again. This time I had chest pain and trouble breathing that started while I was teaching. I also started sweating profusely. I had the same response as last time, just hoping that it would go away. I finally did end up in the hospital again and had another angioplasty. This time the doctors started talking to me about prevention. I started changing my ways, but just could not maintain it.

(continued)

I became complacent and soon I was back to my old habits. Before long, I had one more episode. This time I was on a long drive, heading south to spend the winter. I had been feeling some chest discomfort for a few weeks and had convinced myself that it was acid reflux. I kept thinking that everything would be fine if I could just get where I was going. When the pain became worse I turned the car around and drove home. I don't know what I was thinking. I know that was a risky thing to do, but all I could think about was that I wanted to get home. I was eventually hospitalized again and had another stent.

Believe it or not, I used to give a lecture to my students on the power of denial. I even told them about my first episode and gave them advice not to do what I did. I suppose the message was easier to give others than for me to follow. I should have listened to my own lecture.

I asked my doctor what I should do. He told me to lose twenty pounds and get in an exercise program. It was simple and made a lot of sense. Those direct words made a big impression on me. I can still hear them. I am now exercising, eating well, and taking my medications. My blood pressure and cholesterol are under control. I feel stronger and have more energy.

So now I am taking responsibility. I am determined. I know I have neglected doing what I should have been doing. I have had one too many close calls. I have a spiritual notion that it was not my time. But now I need to keep myself well.

—Richard

CHAPTER 4

Research and Emerging Therapies

Because it's the leading cause of death in America and affects so many people worldwide, heart disease is the subject of billions of dollars of research every year. The print and electronic media know heart disease is a subject people are interested in, too, and, as a result, hardly a day seems to go by without news of promising new research findings. Sometimes—as with the emerging therapies we discuss a bit later in this chapter—these findings hold real hope for heart disease sufferers. Often, however, news stories overstate the significance of newly published research results, sometimes to the surprise and chagrin of the researchers themselves.

Making Sense of New Research

How do you sort out what's important and what's not? By asking yourself a few questions about what you've heard or read:

AT WHAT STAGE IS THE RESEARCH? Research proceeds by stages. The earliest stages often involve laboratory or animal research results and, though these results may be intriguing and published in medical journals, it may be years before the treatment is available for humans—if it ever is.

WHAT KIND OF STUDY IS IT? There are many different kinds of medical research studies, but the most authoritative is the "clinical trial." Clinical trials typically involve large numbers of people who are randomly divided into two groups. One group receives the medication, device, or procedure being tested and the other group receives a harmless alternative. In the best clinical trials, neither the participants nor the lead researchers know who is in which group. This makes it possible to say with some confidence that the results, once the study is completed, are not biased by the natural human tendency to want a positive outcome. By the way, if you have the opportunity, participating in a clinical trial can have real benefits: you're exposed to new treatment ideas early and, because such studies are controlled carefully, you'll receive excellent health care and supervision during the course of the study. Of course, there is the possibility that you'll receive a treatment that has unexpected, and possibly detrimental, effects, so it is important to know that the study was approved by an ethics committee known as an Institutional Review Board. Also, be sure to discuss with your doctor whether participating in clinical trials is possible and appropriate for you.

WHO WAS INVOLVED IN THE STUDY? Some studies involve just a small number of volunteers so that the researchers can understand how the treatment works on people. Others are focused only on certain kinds of people—such as those with a specific kind of heart problem or people in a specific age group. If you're not like those who were studied, the findings may not apply to you.

WHAT ARE THE BENEFITS? It's hard to tell from news reports what the potential benefits of new treatments are for you. Some have been shown to be effective in the laboratory but have yet to be applied to patients. Some eliminate or reduce certain symptoms but have little benefit for you if you don't already experience those symptoms. Still others may truly lower your risk of a heart attack or stroke and increase your chance of living longer.

DO THE BENEFITS OUTWEIGH THE RISKS? Virtually all medical treatments contain some element of risk for some people, so before you begin a new course of treatment, no matter how well publicized, talk with your doctor—especially if the new treatment involves a medication that might interact with others you're taking. What's more, keep in mind that some treatments that at first appear to be beneficial turn out in the end to be detrimental; remember, for example, how our understanding of the risks associated with hormone-replacement therapy has changed as new information has become available. Finally, after you've begun using a new therapy for your heart disease, pay close attention to new research on that treatment; some medications are discovered over time to have unexpected negative side effects for some patients taking them and, as a result, can be taken off the market. Talk with your doctor even if you have not experienced these effects.

Promising New Heart Disease Therapies

Although their findings are not yet featured in the American Heart Association/American College of Cardiology guidelines, many cardiac experts see great promise in several new therapies. Some are still a long way from becoming common practice. Others have been the subject of a lot of good research and, as a result, are already being offered to patients. As research continues on the most successful of these new therapies, the likelihood that they'll be included in the next version of the AHA/ACC guidelines increases. If you have heart disease, or are at risk of heart disease, here are some things you can look forward to in the very near future:

⑦Statins Regardless of Cholesterol Level: Cholesterol Reducers for Everyone

The family of medications called *statins* was first developed to help people with high cholesterol levels. Now researchers are finding that statins may have health benefits even beyond lowering cholesterol. For example, studies show that statins lower the risk that clots will form in the deep veins. For people at risk of heart disease in particular, statins now appear to save lives, above and beyond their cholesterol-lowering action. A study involving more that 20,000 people with a high risk of heart disease found that simvastatin (brand name: Zocor) can reduce the risk of a heart attack or stroke by fully one-third. Now here's the interesting part: this reduction in risk occurred even in patients whose cholesterol levels were normal or low! It is not yet clear exactly what actions of simvastatin made it so beneficial in the study. All we know is that simvastatin appears to save lives. What's more, experts believe that other statins may have the same effect.

There is some suggestion that, in addition to lowering cholesterol, statins may also help to fight inflammation in the blood vessels, and inflammation is increasingly believed to be a cause of heart problems. As things stand now, the only medication the guidelines recommend that every heart disease patient take daily is aspirin. This new research, however, suggests that the guidelines could one day recommend that statin drugs also become a first-line medication for everyone diagnosed with heart disease—regardless of cholesterol levels.

⑦HDL Cholesterol Therapies

Some exciting therapies for the future may be the use of medications that elevate HDL cholesterol levels and clean out the arteries. Some recent studies suggest that this may be just around the corner, and experts are saying that HDL levels are the next big risk factor that will get attention. HDL is thought to work by moving cholesterol from the artery wall back to the liver. The story on HDL became particularly interesting when a group of Italian investigators identified a family that had low HDL levels but no sign of cardiovascular disease. They found that this family had an unusual variant of HDL. A group at the Cleveland Clinic found that giving this special variant to patients (five weekly doses) resulted in a marked improvement in the amount of coronary artery narrowing. Though the study included only forty-seven patients, it elicited quite a lot of interest. The media called the drug "liquid Drano for the arteries." Several other drugs are in development that have the ability to markedly increase HDL levels. This is a very promising area for the future.

★★ Medication-Releasing Stents

Every year, more than half a million Americans undergo angioplasty. It's an operation in which a thin tube is threaded through a patient's blood vessels to permit the insertion of a special balloon that, when inflated, helps widen a coronary artery that has narrowed dangerously and placed the heart at risk. As a treatment, angioplasty is very effective, but its effectiveness can also be short-lived because the artery often narrows again. *Stents* are tiny metal devices invented to keep the artery propped open after angioplasty. But even with stents, the treated arteries of 20 to 30 percent of patients begin closing again within six months.

Now, however, a new kind of stent has been invented that slowly releases a type of drug more commonly used as an immune-system suppressant for patients who have had organ transplants. Research has found that stents that release this kind of drug can keep an artery that had been narrowed by heart disease open long after surgery. In the small number of studies that have been done so far, there were few instances in which patients fitted with these new medication-releasing stents suffered artery reclosure in the short-term. More studies are now being done to investigate the long-term effectiveness of these new stents and what types of medications will work best at keeping the artery open. Experts are still debating who should get this new technology since it is very expensive and does not save lives or prevent heart attacks.

★★★ Implantable Cardiac Defibrillators in Heart Failure or Abnormal Heart Function (ICD Therapy)

Patients who have survived cardiac arrest (when the heart suddenly stops beating) usually owe their lives to a defibrillator, a machine that uses a powerful electric charge to shock the heart into beating again. (You've probably seen those "paddles" used in TV hospital dramas.) But the time in which people whose hearts have stopped can be revived by this treatment is measured in seconds; for too many people, defibrillators aren't available when and where they need them. It's for this reason, for example, that many airlines now carry portable defibrillators and have cabin attendants trained to use them should a passenger be stricken by cardiac arrest while on board. But what if you could carry a defibrillator around with you wherever you go? What if you could have a device implanted in your heart that doesn't just regulate the pace of your heart, the way a pacemaker does, but could also give it a "wake-up call" if needed?

You can. People who are prone to sudden acceleration or irregularity in their heartbeat are at particularly high risk of cardiac arrest. Now, however, defibrillators have been developed that can be implanted directly in the heart, not just to adjust the pace of a racing heart but to "jump-start" that heart if it stops beating altogether. A recent clinical trial involving more than 1,200 patients whose hearts had been weakened by a heart attack found that these patients could be protected from ever experiencing full cardiac arrest through the use of implantable cardiac defibrillators (ICDs). Another large study found that these devices reduced the five-year risk of death in patients with heart failure and weakened hearts by 23 percent. And cardiologists agree that certain patients who have already experienced full cardiac arrest should have an ICD. Having a defibrillator implanted in your heart is a costly procedure, and more research is in progress to determine who is most likely to benefit from it. But if your heart has been weakened by a previous heart attack—that is, if its pumping efficiency is now less than 30 percent, or if you have heart failure and an ejection fraction (the percent of all the blood in your heart that is pumped out with each beat) of less than 35 percent—you should ask your doctor if an ICD is a good option for you.

★★ Cardiac-Resynchronization Therapy for Heart Failure

With each beat, the regions of the heart contract in a way that efficiently pushes the blood forward. For hearts that are damaged, the elegantly choreographed contraction of the heart can be disturbed. This disruption of the normal contraction pattern can lead to inefficient pumping and impair the heart's ability to do its job. To address this problem, doctors are using a new type of pacemaker that can restore the normal contraction pattern and enhance the heart's performance. This special pacemaker seems to be highly effective in patients with heart failure and evidence of an abnormal contraction pattern—something that is usually indicated by a specific pattern on the electrocardiogram. The early studies have been very encouraging, and experience with this device is growing.

⑦Gene Therapy

The genes we inherit from our parents can affect profoundly our vulnerability to certain diseases and our ability to combat them. That's why, for example, some diseases are more common in some families than in others. But gene research has begun to give us the tools to alter some of these predispositions and to more effectively respond to disease when it arises. Of course, many of the risk factors associated with heart disease aren't caused by heredity but rather by the way we choose to live our lives. Still, gene therapy holds great promise for treating some kinds of heart disease—especially in cases where much of the problem is caused by diminished blood flow to the heart. For example, researchers have designed new gene-altering drugs that improve blood flow to damaged areas of the heart by triggering the growth of new blood vessels, thus decreasing significantly the severity of symptoms in some heart disease patients. This work is very new, and we don't know enough yet about the long-term effect of therapies like these. We don't even know with certainty whether such results can be reproduced reliably in other patients. But initial results are promising, and treatments like these may be available for wider public use soon.

⑦Anti-Inflammatory Markers and Medications

As we've noted elsewhere in this book, research suggests that blood vessel inflammation may be a more important cause of heart disease than even cholesterol. This may well be why aspirin, an anti-inflammatory, is so effective against the disease. Researchers are looking closely at something called "C-reactive protein," a marker in the blood that signals inflammation, to determine whether it might be used to diagnose and evaluate one's risk of heart trouble. This protein was discovered more than seventy years ago, but only recently have scientists determined its connection to heart disease.

Experts from the American Heart Association and the Centers for Disease Control and Prevention have concluded that a high C-reactive protein level in the blood does indeed appear to be an important risk factor for heart problems. Studies show that people with high C-reactive protein levels have a much higher risk of heart attack, sudden death, and narrowing of the arteries than people with low levels. Recent work suggests that C-reactive protein may be an even stronger predictor of heart problems than LDL (bad) cholesterol. Therefore, people who do not have heart disease may have their C-reactive protein level measured to assess their heart disease risk. This protein should be measured with a "high-sensitivity" test, which is different from the way that it was traditionally measured. This newer test can detect much lower levels of C-reactive protein.

The AHA and CDC recommend that people who have heart disease be treated aggressively for their condition, using the key strategies mentioned in this book, regardless of their C-reactive protein levels. These experts do suggest that this test can be used along with cholesterol and other risk factors to determine a person's risk of heart disease. If you have had a recent heart attack it is better to wait six or eight weeks before measuring it. As the role of C-reactive protein in heart disease continues to be studied, we may see an increase in the use of anti-inflammatory medications to prevent and treat heart disease. An ongoing trial is even assessing the effectiveness of statins in treating an elevated C-reactive protein level. For now, however, there is no specific treatment for this condition.

CHAPTER 5

Staying Well and Prepared

As I said at the outset, the whole point of this book is to equip you with the knowledge you need to take charge of your heart disease. Modern medicine can't cure you of this disease—not yet, at least—but it certainly can help you live with it, and live well.

Look at it this way: staying well and prepared is your job and, like any job, it will take some work. In this chapter we look at some of that work and provide guidance on how to monitor your heart's health, how to guard against two other health issues that can affect your heart's health profoundly, how to make the most of your visits to the doctor, and how to be prepared for any possible event.

Monitoring Your Heart's Health

Are the Key Strategies Working?
The most important thing you can do to monitor your heart's health is to keep track of your progress in achieving the goals of the key strategies. On a regular basis, you should ask yourself:

1. Is my blood pressure at my target level?

2. Is my cholesterol at my target level?

3. Is my blood sugar at my target level?

4. Is my weight at my target level?

5. Am I getting enough of the right kind of exercise for my heart?

6. Am I taking the right medications, and taking them correctly?

To help you keep track of your progress toward these goals, we've provided a number of detailed logs and checklists in the Appendices. Make a habit of using them. If you notice that despite your best efforts you're not reaching your goals, see your doctor and work out a new plan for reaching them. Remember, every person with heart disease is different; sometimes it takes a bit of trial and error to put together a therapy plan that works for you. But unless you're keeping track, you won't know how you're doing.

How's My Heart Doing?

In a sense, keeping track of your key strategy levels and goals is an indirect way of checking on your heart. Your progress toward each target provides a piece of information from which you, and your doctor, can get a sense of where you are in your recovery program. But the most direct and important measure of the health of your heart is the extent to which it affects your day-to-day activities. To determine the extent to which your heart disease affects the quality of your life, take the short Seattle Angina Questionnaire that's included in Appendix C of this book. It's a reliable tool doctors use to assess how heart disease is affecting the lives of their patients and it can be a revealing tool for you, too. It may also be a useful way to convey to your doctor how your symptoms are affecting you.

Doctors refer to heart disease in a patient as being either "stable" or "unstable." If your heart disease is stable, you may experience one or more of the following symptoms when you exert yourself:

- chest tightness or chest, jaw, or arm discomfort (angina);

- unusual breathlessness;

- fast or irregular heartbeat (palpitations);

- sweatiness;

- dizziness or light-headedness;

- swelling in the feet or ankles; and/or

- fatigue.

In the case of stable heart disease, these symptoms are typically mild, are fairly predictable, go away promptly when you rest or take nitroglycerin pills or sprays, and have not worsened with time. A word of caution, though: some heart disease sufferers experience none of these symptoms. If you are one of them, you'll want to work closely with your doctor to try to identify your own early warning signs.

If symptoms like these are new to you, are getting worse, or are occurring unpredictably, your heart disease may have become unstable, and that's serious. You should contact your doctor right away. If these symptoms have worsened very quickly, or have become severe, you should go to an emergency room instead. And if you suddenly experience a severe, crushing chest pain that is accompanied by sweating, light-headedness, nausea, or breathlessness and lasts more than five minutes, you may be having a heart attack. Seek emergency medical assistance immediately.

Guarding Against Other Health Risks

Elsewhere in this book I've discussed medical conditions that increase the risk and potential severity of heart disease, including high blood pressure, diabetes, and high cholesterol. More recently, however, two other medical conditions have been shown to increase your risk of heart disease: flu and depression. Research on the effects of these conditions is still emerging, but you should know about them.

The Flu

Each year, new strains of the influenza, or flu, virus appear, and each year researchers acquire early samples of the new strains to create vaccines against the disease. The fact that this virus keeps altering itself is one reason why the vaccine you get one year won't protect you in the next. Do flu vaccines guarantee you won't get infected? No, but they're remarkably effective, lowering your chances of getting this year's flu by anywhere between 30 and 90 percent. In adults over the age of 65, flu shots lower the chance of getting pneumonia and being hospitalized by 50 to 60 percent and provide an 80 percent better chance of living through the flu season.

More important for our purposes here, one recent study of more than 200 people who had a previous heart attack found that getting a flu shot lowered their risk of having a second heart attack during that flu season by 67 percent. Yet another study found that a flu shot can lower the risk of stroke by 50 to 60 percent. It is not yet clear exactly how a flu shot may prevent heart attacks. One theory holds that getting sick with the flu contributes to heart attacks by causing inflammation in the area around atherosclerotic plaques in the blood vessels. Another theory suggests that the flu illness thickens the blood and therefore encourages the buildup of clots. It could also be that the flu influences the composition of the blood, which, in turn, increases the risk of a heart attack. Still, whatever the precise mechanism, the fact that a therapy so routine and safe might also prevent heart attacks and strokes suggests that everybody with heart disease should get an annual flu shot.

The Centers for Disease Control and Prevention has identified five groups of people who are at particular risk from the flu and who, therefore, should get a flu shot before or at the beginning of each flu season:

- people age 50 or older;

- residents of nursing homes and other care facilities that house people with long-term illnesses;

- anyone six months or older who has a chronic heart or lung condition, including asthma;

- anyone six months or older who needs regular medical care or has been in a hospital because of metabolic diseases (like diabetes), chronic kidney disease, or weakened immune system (including immune system problems caused by medicine or by infection with human immunodeficiency virus [HIV]); and

- women who will be more than three months pregnant during the flu season.

Depression

Centuries ago, before the advent of modern medicine, it was thought that the heart was the seat of our emotions. And while that romantic notion lingers in music and literature, we now know that emotion is more often than not controlled by the action of various neurotransmitter chemicals in the brain. But in at least one respect science is also beginning to demonstrate a dual link between the heart and emotion. It is this: heart disease can cause depression, and depression can cause heart disease.

In the first instance, this is hardly surprising. The sudden sense of vulnerability and mortality brought on by a heart attack or a diagnosis of heart disease can, and does, cause emotional distress in many people. As many as two-thirds of people who have had a heart attack report symptoms of depression, and up to 20 percent of heart disease patients who have never had a heart attack report feeling depressed.

This alone would be troubling, but there is another side to this story. It turns out that people who are depressed are 70 percent more likely to develop heart disease. What's more, people who have heart disease and are depressed have a three or four times greater risk of dying from a heart attack, and patients with depression who have survived one heart attack are more likely than non-depressed patients to have future heart problems.

The reasons for this are not entirely clear. It may be that depression increases the risk of heart disease by causing a rapid heart rate, high blood pressure, irregular heart rhythms, faster blood-clotting time, and higher levels of insulin and cholesterol in the blood. But it's also possible that people who are depressed tend to exercise less, smoke more, and eat unhealthy foods—all behaviors that can increase the risk for heart disease.

Whatever the reason, there's good news: the vast majority of people suffering from depression can be treated successfully. But this only works if they seek help, and many don't. Indeed, many people don't know the signs of depression, in part because some of the signs of depression are fairly commonplace. As a general rule, if you have five of the following symptoms and they last for more than two weeks, you should talk to your doctor about depression:

1. a persistent sad or "empty" mood;

2. loss of interest or pleasure in activities, including sex;

3. difficulty concentrating, remembering, or making decisions;

4. feelings of guilt, worthlessness, or helplessness;

5. decreased energy, fatigue, or a feeling of being "slowed down";

6. insomnia, early-morning wakening, or oversleeping;

7. loss of appetite with weight loss, or weight gain;

8. thoughts of death or suicide or suicide attempts;

9. irritability;

10. chronic aches and pains that don't respond to treatment; and

11. excessive crying.

In the past, the depression medications that were available could not be prescribed for patients with heart disease because they had the potential to cause additional heart problems, but that's changed. Today, newer antidepressants are not only safe but highly effective, improving the symptoms of up to 75 percent of the patients with heart disease who take them.

In addition, other forms of therapy, including cognitive behavioral therapy (CBT), which stresses changing or adjusting to stressful parts of your environment, individual counseling, and support-group counseling have all been demonstrated to be effective for alleviating depression. In fact, research suggests that CBT or individual therapy, undertaken in conjunction with medication, is even more effective at relieving depression than medication alone.

Finally, an important caution: the professional treating your depression probably won't be the doctor treating your heart disease, and there is always a possibility that the drugs recommended by one may interact with those prescribed by the other. Make sure all your doctors and health care providers know what medications you're taking and why you're taking them.

Making the Most of Your Doctor's Appointment

Although doctors are trained to make diagnoses from sometimes limited clues, they're not clairvoyant; they can't read your mind or your body. They can order an array of tests to strengthen their diagnosis (see Appendix E, "Tests and Medical Procedures"), but their most important source of information is you. The more information you can give your doctors about the state of your health, the more likely you are to get the best possible care. This is more important today than ever, as changes in the structure of our health care system have made doctors increasingly pressed for time. There are three things you can do to make your trip to the doctor successful:

1. Make a List

It can be hard to remember all the things you want to talk to the doctor about once you're in the examining room, so make a list before you go, and include:

- symptoms you've experienced, especially those that have changed or are new;

- major health events that have taken place recently, especially if they were treated by someone else;

- problems with or side effects from any medications you're taking;

- concerns you have about your ongoing care;

- specific questions you have about upcoming tests or procedures (see Appendix E: "Tests and Medical Procedures"); and

- travel plans you have for the near future.

2. Be Honest

You needn't be embarrassed or afraid to mention anything to your doctor that troubles you, whether it's a symptom, a side effect, or difficulty sticking with a diet or exercise regimen. Your doctor has only one concern, and that's to help you get better. Try to be specific and direct when you describe your concerns or complaints; that will make the doctor's job easier and make it more likely your condition will be correctly diagnosed and treated. For example, rather than saying you have had a problem for a while, try to pinpoint the number of days, etc.

3. Take Your Medications with You

In this age of specialists, you're likely to have several different doctors, each of whom may be prescribing medications for you. In order to protect you against harmful drug interactions, each doctor needs to know all of the drugs you are taking, including over-the-counter drugs and supplements. Take the containers with you (probably the best approach) or make a list of the types of medications you're taking and the dosages. In fact, it's a good idea to carry this list with you at all times in case of emergencies. If you purchase all your medications at one pharmacy, they may be able to print out a complete list for you.

Advance Planning

This book is about taking charge of heart disease, but it is also about knowledge and planning. If you have heart disease (or even if you do not) there may ultimately come a day when you are so ill that you can no longer participate in the important decisions relating to your care.

Even as the information in this book helps you beat heart disease, it is important to plan for the possibility of being so sick that you cannot convey your preferences about the kind of medical treatment that you receive. To prepare for this type of situation, the kinds of questions that you want to answer for yourself include:

- How do I want to be treated at the end of my life?

- Are there particular treatments that I would or would not want?

- If I could not make health care decisions for myself, is there somebody in particular whom I would want to make those decisions on my behalf?

- Just in case, what should I do to ensure that my affairs are in order?

Your preferences for care—should such a time like this occur—may depend on a number of factors, including: your likelihood of a meaningful recovery; your personal attitude toward life, death, and illness; how you value independence and control; and any religious or moral convictions you may have.

No one lives forever. This book is about helping you to live a long and productive life, but ultimately we will all face difficult decisions about our care during our last days. While these decisions are your own to make, you will want to discuss with your loved ones your decisions and your reasons for making them. This will help prevent any confusion about what your end-of-life care should be.

Once you have made decisions about your end-of-life preferences, you should let your doctor know. Your decisions can then be included in your medical record and be made available to any health care team that looks after you in the future. This type of planning does *not* mean that people will give up on you; what it does mean is that you will maintain control over how you are treated even when you can no longer participate in those decisions.

You can also specify your end-of-life preferences in detail, in the form of *advance directives*, which are legal documents that come in two types:

1. *Living will.* A document that states your specific instructions on the type of medical care you would like to receive in the event that you are unable to speak for yourself because of serious illness.

2. *Medical power of attorney.* A document that names a person whom you entrust to make medical care decisions on your behalf in the event that you are unable to make these decisions for yourself.

Since different states treat these documents differently, you should ask your doctor about how advance directives and end-of-life planning work where you live. You should also know that you can change your end-of-life preferences any time you wish. Simply keep your documents and your doctor up to date with any changes.

Conclusion

By reading this book, you have already started to make choices about the care of your current condition so that you can optimize your health outcomes over the course of your life. In the new age of medicine we will see the best results in patients who take responsibility and take control of their care. I urge you to be actively involved in your care—to know what strategies are best for you—and to take charge of your heart health.

APPENDICES

Quick Guide to Heart Disease Treatments

Many treatments are commonly recommended for fighting heart disease. Some therapies have been shown by solid science to have true benefit for the heart. Others need to be more researched before we can know if there is any effect at all. Still others have been shown to have no effect, or even to be harmful. This Quick Guide uses symbols to summarize what we know so far about the usefulness of the treatments, listed below, for fighting heart disease.

Proven benefit ★★★	Probable benefit ★★	Possible benefit ★	Unclear effect ⑦	No effect ⊘	Harmful ①
Controlling blood pressure	Eating fatty fish	Eating fruits and vegetables	Eating smaller, more frequent meals	Taking vitamin E	Possibly hormone replacement therapy
Managing cholesterol	Cardiac resynchronization therapy for specific groups with heart failure	Eating whole grains	Eating garlic		
Exercising		Continuing to drink moderate amounts of alcohol	Drinking black tea		
Optimizing weight		Consuming fiber	Starting to drink moderate amounts of alcohol if you were not a drinker before		
Watching sugars		Consuming nuts			
Not smoking		Stress reduction	Taking folic acid or B vitamins		
Taking aspirin			Taking multivitamins		
Taking a beta-blocker			Taking herbal medicines		
Taking an ACE inhibitor					
ICD Therapy for specific groups					

Tools for Success

The forms and tables below and on the following pages are tools that you can use to keep yourself on track for optimal heart health.

- *Just-after-a-Heart-Attack Checklist*
- *My Healthy Heart Log*
- *My Blood Pressure Log*
- *My Cholesterol Log*
- *My Weight Log*
- *My Exercise Log*
- *My Sugars Log*

The first two tools can help you monitor your overall heart health care. The others are designed to help you implement specific key strategies for fighting heart disease.

Not everybody needs to use every tool to ensure he or she is getting the best care for their heart. However, if there is a key strategy that you are struggling to put into action, you may find it helpful to use the appropriate tool to plan your approach and chart your progress. You may also choose to adapt any of these tools to fit your own specific needs.

Just-After-a-Heart-Attack Checklist

	Yes	No	N/A	Notes
Am I taking an aspirin once a day?	❏	❏	❏	
(Or, if I cannot take aspirin for a medical reason, am I taking clopidogrel once a day?)	❏	❏	❏	
If I am taking aspirin, am I also taking clopidogrel once a day up to 9 months after my heart attack?	❏	❏	❏	
Am I taking a beta-blocker?	❏	❏	❏	
If my LDL cholesterol level was over 100 mg/dL by the time I left the hospital, am I taking a statin?	❏	❏	❏	
Am I taking an ACE inhibitor?	❏	❏	❏	
Am I taking an aldosterone antagonist if I do not have renal dysfunction or high potassium levels, am taking an ACE inhibitor, have an ejection fraction of less than or equal to 40%, and have symptomatic heart failure?	❏	❏	❏	

My Healthy Heart Log

	month: _____ year: _____			month: _____ year: _____			month: _____ year: _____		
	Yes	No	If no, do I have an action plan?	Yes	No	If no, do I have an action plan?	Yes	No	If no, do I have an action plan?
Do I take the following medications?									
▪ an aspirin every day	☐	☐	☐	☐	☐	☐	☐	☐	☐
▪ a beta-blocker every day	☐	☐	☐	☐	☐	☐	☐	☐	☐
▪ an ACE inhibitor every day	☐	☐	☐	☐	☐	☐	☐	☐	☐
Is my blood pressure less than 140/90 (or 130/85 if I have heart failure, or 130/80 if I have diabetes)?	☐	☐	☐	☐	☐	☐	☐	☐	☐
Is my LDL cholesterol less than 100?	☐	☐	☐	☐	☐	☐	☐	☐	☐
Do I exercise at least 30 minutes per day, at least 3 times per week?	☐	☐	☐	☐	☐	☐	☐	☐	☐
Is my weight at a level where my BMI is 19 to 25?*	☐	☐	☐	☐	☐	☐	☐	☐	☐

*You can determine your body mass index (BMI) using the charts on page 64.

My Healthy Heart Log

	month: _____ year: _____			month: _____ year: _____			month: _____ year: _____		
	Yes	No	If no, do I have an action plan?	Yes	No	If no, do I have an action plan?	Yes	No	If no, do I have an action plan?
If I have diabetes, is my HbA1c below 7%?	☐	☐	☐	☐	☐	☐	☐	☐	☐
Am I a non-smoker?	☐	☐	☐	☐	☐	☐	☐	☐	☐

My Blood Pressure Log

Goals:

Systolic Blood Pressure (SNP) < 140 mmHg

Diastolic Blood Pressure (DBP) < 90 mmHg

Goals for People with Heart or Kidney Failure

SBP < 130 mmHg

DBP < 85 mmHg

Goals for People with Diabetes

SBP < 130 mmHg

DBP < 80 mmHg

***You should have your blood pressure checked every 1 to 3 months after starting a new therapy. After your blood pressure has been at goal and stable, you should have your blood pressure checked every 3 to 6 months and every time you see a doctor.

Date	SBP	DBP	Blood pressure–lowering medication(s) I was on when my BP was checked				Notes
			medication & dose	*medication & dose*	*medication & dose*	*medication & dose*	

Example of how to use your Blood Pressure Log

Goals:

Systolic Blood Pressure (SNP) < 140 mmHg
Diastolic Blood Pressure (DBP) < 90 mmHg

Goals for People with Heart or Kidney Failure

SBP < 130 mmHg
DBP < 85 mmHg

Goals for People with Diabetes

SBP < 130 mmHg
DBP < 80 mmHg

***You should have your blood pressure checked every 1 to 3 months after starting a new therapy. After your blood pressure has been at goal and stable, you should have your blood pressure checked every 3 to 6 months and every time you see a doctor.

Date	SBP	DBP	Blood pressure–lowering medication(s) I was on when my BP was checked				Notes
			medication & dose	*medication & dose*	*medication & dose*	*medication & dose*	
May 2, '04	175	100	HCTZ 25 mg/day	atenolol 50 mg/day			continuing low salt
June 4, '04	170	95	"	"	ramipril 10 mg/day		got cough (ramipril)
July 3, '04	160	90	"	"	losartan 50 mg/day		no side effects
Aug. 10, '04	155	90	"	"	"		"

My Cholesterol Log

Primary Goal:
LDL cholesterol < 100 mg/dL

Secondary Goals
HDL cholesterol > 40 mg/dL
Total cholesterol < 200 mg/dL
Triglycerides < 200mg/dL

***You should have your fasting cholesterol and triglyceride levels measured every 6 weeks after starting a new therapy, and then every 4 to 6 months afterward.

Date of test	Fasting		Cholesterol			Triglycerides	Cholesterol-lowering medication(s) I was on when my cholesterol was measured		Notes
	yes	no	LDL	HDL	Total		medication & dose	medication & dose	
	☐	☐							
	☐	☐							
	☐	☐							
	☐	☐							
	☐	☐							
	☐	☐							
	☐	☐							

Example of how to use your Cholesterol Log

Primary Goal:
LDL cholesterol < 100 mg/dL

Secondary Goals
HDL cholesterol > 40 mg/dL
Total cholesterol < 200 mg/dL
Triglycerides < 200mg/dL

***You should have your fasting cholesterol and triglyceride levels measured every 6 weeks after starting a new therapy, and then every 4 to 6 months afterwards.

Date of test	Fasting		Cholesterol			Triglycerides	Cholesterol-lowering medication(s) I was on when my cholesterol was measured		Notes
	yes	no	LDL	HDL	Total		medication & dose	medication & dose	
May 3, '04	☑	☐	145	20	245	400	atorvastatin 10 mg/day		on low-fat diet
Jun 14, '04	☐	☑	140	22	239	385	atorvastatin 20 mg/day		no med side effects
Jul 26, '04	☑	☐	120	25	204	295	atorvastatin 40 mg/day	gemfibrozil 600 mg 2×/day	no med side effects

My Weight Log

Primary Goal: Body Mass Index (BMI) between 18.5 and 24.9.

My height = _____ inches.

For my BMI to be between 18.5 and 24.9, my weight should ideally be between _____ and _____ pounds.*

Secondary Goals If your BMI is 25 or more, your waistline should be 40 inches or less if you are male, 35 inches or less if you are female.

*To calculate your ideal weight range, use the BMI calculation table at the end of the Optimize Your Weight section on page 64.

Date	Weight	Waistline	Therapies I was on when my weight was checked			Notes
			diet	exercise	medication & dose	

Example of how to use your Weight Log

Primary Goal: ⎰ Body Mass Index (BMI) between 18.5 and 24.9.

My height = _____ inches.

For my BMI to be between 18.5 and 24.9, my weight should ideally be between _____ and _____ pounds.*

Secondary Goals ⎱ If your BMI is 25 or more, your waistline should be 40 inches or less if you are male, 35 inches or less if you are female.

*To calculate your ideal weight range, use the BMI calculation table at the end of the Optimize Your Weight section on page 64.

Date	Weight	Waistline	Therapies I was on when my weight was checked				Notes
			diet	exercise	medication & dose		
May 3, '04	185 lbs	35 inches	2,200 cal per day, low fat	20-min. walk. 2 per week			
June 14, '04	183 lbs	34 inches	2,200 cal per day, low fat	20-min. walk. 3 per week			

My Exercise Log

Check off the days of the week you completed the program

Week	Activity Program			Su	M	Tu	W	Th	F	Sa	Notes
	Warm-up	Exercise	Cool-down								
				☐	☐	☐	☐	☐	☐	☐	
				☐	☐	☐	☐	☐	☐	☐	
				☐	☐	☐	☐	☐	☐	☐	
				☐	☐	☐	☐	☐	☐	☐	
				☐	☐	☐	☐	☐	☐	☐	
				☐	☐	☐	☐	☐	☐	☐	
				☐	☐	☐	☐	☐	☐	☐	
				☐	☐	☐	☐	☐	☐	☐	
				☐	☐	☐	☐	☐	☐	☐	
				☐	☐	☐	☐	☐	☐	☐	
				☐	☐	☐	☐	☐	☐	☐	
				☐	☐	☐	☐	☐	☐	☐	
				☐	☐	☐	☐	☐	☐	☐	
				☐	☐	☐	☐	☐	☐	☐	
				☐	☐	☐	☐	☐	☐	☐	

Example of a Walking Program

Goals: How often: Exercise at least 3 times per week   How long: Spend 30 to 60 minutes briskly walking each time you exercise

Week	Activity Program			Check off the days of the week you completed the program							Notes
	Warm-up walk easily for…	*Exercise* walk briskly for…	*Cool-down* walk slowly for…	Su	M	Tu	W	Th	F	Sa	
1	5 min.	5 min.	5 min.	❏	❏	❏	❏	❏	❏	❏	
2	5 min.	7 min.	5 min.	❏	❏	❏	❏	❏	❏	❏	
3	5 min.	9 min.	5 min.	❏	❏	❏	❏	❏	❏	❏	
4	5 min.	11 min.	5 min.	❏	❏	❏	❏	❏	❏	❏	
5	5 min.	13 min.	5 min.	❏	❏	❏	❏	❏	❏	❏	
6	5 min.	15 min.	5 min.	❏	❏	❏	❏	❏	❏	❏	
7	5 min.	18 min.	5 min.	❏	❏	❏	❏	❏	❏	❏	
8	5 min.	20 min.	5 min.	❏	❏	❏	❏	❏	❏	❏	
9	5 min.	23 min.	5 min.	❏	❏	❏	❏	❏	❏	❏	
10	5 min.	26 min.	5 min.	❏	❏	❏	❏	❏	❏	❏	
11	5 min.	28 min.	5 min.	❏	❏	❏	❏	❏	❏	❏	
12	5 min.	30 min.	5 min.	❏	❏	❏	❏	❏	❏	❏	
13	5 min.	30 or 33 min.	5 min.	❏	❏	❏	❏	❏	❏	❏	
14	5 min.	30 or 36 min.	5 min.	❏	❏	❏	❏	❏	❏	❏	
15	5 min.	*and so on…*	5 min.	❏	❏	❏	❏	❏	❏	❏	

Adapted from the National Heart, Lung, and Blood Institute *Guide to Physical Activity*, October 2000.

Example of a Jogging Program

Goals: How often: Exercise at least 3 times per week   How long: Spend 20 to 60 minutes jogging each time you exercise

Week	Warm-up		Exercise	Cool-down		Check off the days of the week you completed the program						
	Activity Program					Su	M	Tu	W	Th	F	Sa
	walk easily for …	stretch & limber up for …	then …	walk slowly for …	stretch for …							
1	5 min.	2 min.	walk 10 min.	3 min.	2 min.	❏	❏	❏	❏	❏	❏	❏
2	5 min.	2 min.	walk 5 min., jog 1 min., walk 5 min, jog 1 min.	3 min.	2 min.	❏	❏	❏	❏	❏	❏	❏
3	5 min.	2 min.	walk 5 min., jog 3 min., walk 5 min., jog 3 min.	3 min.	2 min.	❏	❏	❏	❏	❏	❏	❏
4	5 min.	2 min.	walk 4 min., jog 5 min., walk 4 min., jog 5 min.	3 min.	2 min.	❏	❏	❏	❏	❏	❏	❏
5	5 min.	2 min.	walk 4 min., jog 5 min., walk 4 min., jog 5 min.	3 min.	2 min.	❏	❏	❏	❏	❏	❏	❏
6	5 min.	2 min.	walk 4 min., jog 6 min., walk 4 min., jog 6 min.	3 min.	2 min.	❏	❏	❏	❏	❏	❏	❏
7	5 min.	2 min.	walk 4 min., jog 7 min., walk 4 min., jog 7 min.	3 min.	2 min.	❏	❏	❏	❏	❏	❏	❏
8	5 min.	2 min.	walk 4 min., jog 8 min., walk 4 min., jog 8 min.	3 min.	2 min.	❏	❏	❏	❏	❏	❏	❏
9	5 min.	2 min.	walk 4 min., jog 9 min., walk 4 min., jog 9 min.	3 min.	2 min.	❏	❏	❏	❏	❏	❏	❏

Example of a Jogging Program (continued)

Goals: How often: Exercise at least 3 times per week   How long: Spend 20 to 60 minutes jogging each time you exercise

Week	Warm-up		Exercise	Cool-down		Su	M	Tu	W	Th	F	Sa
	walk easily for…	stretch & limber up for…	then…	walk slowly for…	stretch for…	Check off the days of the week you completed the program						
10	5 min.	2 min.	walk 4 min., jog 13 min.	3 min.	2 min.	❑	❑	❑	❑	❑	❑	❑
11	5 min.	2 min.	walk 4 min., jog 15 min.	3 min.	2 min.	❑	❑	❑	❑	❑	❑	❑
12	5 min.	2 min.	walk 4 min., jog 17 min.	3 min.	2 min.	❑	❑	❑	❑	❑	❑	❑
13	5 min.	2 min.	walk 2 min., jog slowly 2 min., jog 17 min.	3 min.	2 min.	❑	❑	❑	❑	❑	❑	❑
14	5 min.	2 min.	walk 1 min., jog slowly 3 min., jog 17 min.	3 min.	2 min.	❑	❑	❑	❑	❑	❑	❑
15	5 min.	2 min.	jog slowly 3 min., jog 17 min.	3 min.	2 min.	❑	❑	❑	❑	❑	❑	❑
16	5 min.	2 min.	jog slowly 2 min., jog 18 min.	3 min.	2 min.	❑	❑	❑	❑	❑	❑	❑
17	5 min.	2 min.	*build up to a 20-min. jog or as desired…*	3 min.	2 min.	❑	❑	❑	❑	❑	❑	❑

Adapted from the National Heart, Lung, and Blood Institute *Guide to Physical Activity*, October 2000.

My Sugars Log

Primary Goal: Hemoglobin (Hb) A1c < 7%

Secondary Goals $\begin{cases} \text{Fasting blood glucose level 80 to 120 mg/dL} \\ \text{Non-fasting blood glucose level 100 to} \\ \text{140 mg/dL} \end{cases}$

Every person with **heart disease** should have their fasting blood glucose checked at least every 2 years.

- If you have **diabetes** and are *not on insulin*, you should check your blood glucose a few times per week, and your HbA1c every 3 months.
- If you have **diabetes** and are *on insulin*, you should check your blood glucose 3 to 4 times a day, and your HbA1c every 3 months.

Date	Time	When the test was done in relation to eating		Glucose level	HbA1c level	Diabetes medication(s) I was regularly taking when my blood glucose or HbA1c was measured		
		just before a meal or after a fast	just after a meal			*medication & dose*	*medication & dose*	*medication & dose*
		❏	❏					
		❏	❏					
		❏	❏					
		❏	❏					
		❏	❏					
		❏	❏					
		❏	❏					

Example of how to use your Sugars Log

Date	Time	When the test was done in relation to eating		Glucose level	HbA1c level	Diabetes medication(s) I was regularly taking when my blood glucose or HbA1c was measured		
		just before a meal or after a fast	just after a meal			*medication & dose*	*medication & dose*	*medication & dose*
5/4/04	10 A.M.	☑	❏	185	6.5	R insulin 12U at meals	NPH insulin 24U at bed	glyburide 3 mg/day
5/4/04	9 P.M.	☑	❏	135		"	"	"

Seattle Angina Questionnaire

This survey, developed by Dr. John Spertus, is designed to help doctors and patients better understand how heart disease symptoms (specifically angina or chest discomfort) affect quality of life. You and your doctor can use this survey to gain a better sense of how heart disease is affecting your life and how this may change over time. For more information about the Seattle Angina Questionnaire, you can check out www.cvoutcomes.org.

1. The following is a list of activities that people often do during the week. Although for some people with several medical problems it is difficult to determine what it is that limits them, please go over the activities listed below and indicate how much limitation you have had due to chest pain, chest tightness, or angina over the past 4 weeks.

activity	severely limited	moder- ately limited	some- what limited	a little limited	not limited	limited, or did not do for other reasons
dressing yourself	❏	❏	❏	❏	❏	❏

activity	severely limited	moder-ately limited	some-what limited	a little limited	not limited	limited, or did not do for other reasons
walking indoors on level ground	❑	❑	❑	❑	❑	❑
showering	❑	❑	❑	❑	❑	❑
climbing a hill or a flight of stairs without stopping	❑	❑	❑	❑	❑	❑
gardening, vacuuming, or carrying groceries	❑	❑	❑	❑	❑	❑
walking more than a block at a brisk pace	❑	❑	❑	❑	❑	❑
running or jogging	❑	❑	❑	❑	❑	❑
lifting or moving heavy objects (e.g., furniture, children)	❑	❑	❑	❑	❑	❑
participating in strenuous sports (e.g., swimming, tennis)	❑	❑	❑	❑	❑	❑

2. Compared with 4 weeks ago, how often do you have chest pain, chest tightness, or angina when doing your most strenuous level of activity? I have had chest pain, chest tightness, or angina . . .

much more often	slightly more often	about the same	slightly less often	much less often
❑	❑	❑	❑	❑

3. Over the past 4 weeks, on average, how many times have you had chest pain, chest tightness, or angina? I get chest pain, chest tightness, or angina . . .

4 or more times per day	1–3 times per day	3 or more times per week but not every day	1–2 times per week	less than once per week	none over the past 4 weeks
❑	❑	❑	❑	❑	❑

4. Over the past 4 weeks, on average, how many times have you had to take nitros (nitroglycerin tablets) for your chest pain, chest tightness, or angina? I take nitros . . .

4 or more times per day	1–3 times per day	3 or more times per week but not every day	1–2 times per week	less than once per week	none over the past 4 weeks
❑	❑	❑	❑	❑	❑

5. How bothersome is it for you to take your pills for chest pain, chest tightness, or angina as prescribed?

very bothersome	moderately bothersome	somewhat bothersome	a little bothersome	not bothersome at all	my doctor has not prescribed pills
❑	❑	❑	❑	❑	❑

6. How satisfied are you that everything possible is being done to treat your chest pain, chest tightness, or angina?

not satisfied at all	mostly dissatisfied	somewhat satisfied	mostly satisfied	highly satisfied
❑	❑	❑	❑	❑

7. How satisfied are you with the explanations your doctor has given you about your chest pain, chest tightness, or angina?

not satisfied at all	mostly dissatisfied	somewhat satisfied	mostly satisfied	highly satisfied
❑	❑	❑	❑	❑

8. Overall, how satisfied are you with the current treatment of your chest pain, chest tightness, or angina?

not satisfied at all	mostly dissatisfied	somewhat satisfied	mostly satisfied	highly satisfied
❑	❑	❑	❑	❑

9. Over the past 4 weeks, how much has your chest pain, chest tightness, or angina interfered with your enjoyment of life?

it has severely limited my enjoyment of life	it has moderately limited my enjoyment of life	it has slightly limited my enjoyment of life	it has barely limited my enjoyment of life	it has not limited my enjoyment of life
❑	❑	❑	❑	❑

10. If you had to spend the rest of your life with your chest pain, chest tightness, or angina the way it is right now, how would you feel about this?

not satisfied at all	mostly dissatisfied	somewhat satisfied	mostly satisfied	highly satisfied
❑	❑	❑	❑	❑

11. How often do you worry that you may have a heart attack or die suddenly?

I can't stop worrying about it	I often think or worry about it	I occasionally worry about it	I rarely think or worry about it	I never think or worry about it
❑	❑	❑	❑	❑

Drug Interactions

Thanks to advances in medical science, we now have many medications available to help people with heart disease lower their risk of having future heart problems. While taking advantage of the benefits these medications have to offer, it is important to keep in mind the possible interactions your medications can have with each other, with certain foods, or with non-prescription medications you may be taking.

Below is an outline of some drug interactions to watch out for. Some interactions may be more serious than others, so if you are taking any of the drug combinations listed below, you should learn more about the potential interactions by discussing them with your doctor or pharmacist.

Note that this outline should be used only as a guide since it is not a complete list or description of all the possible interactions the medications below may have with other things you may be taking. You should discuss with your doctor or pharmacist any concerns about possible interactions with any of your medications.

Blood Thinners	
The drug below . . .	**may interact with . . .**

aspirin	another blood thinner
	certain anti-inflammatory medications
	  (e.g., ibuprofen, naproxen)
	certain herbals: dong quai, feverfew, garlic,
	  ginger, ginkgo biloba, kava

clopidogrel	another blood thinner
	certain anti-inflammatory medications
	  (e.g., ibuprofen, naproxen)
	certain herbals: dong quai, feverfew, garlic,
	  ginger, ginkgo biloba, kava

warfarin	another blood thinner
	certain antidepressants: fluoxetine,
	  fluvoxamine, nefazodone, sertraline
	certain anti-inflammatory medications
	  (e.g., ibuprofen, naproxen)
	certain antivirals: ritonavir, saquinavir
	certain herbals: dong quai, feverfew, garlic,
	  ginger, ginkgo biloba, kava
	certain antibiotics: ciprofloxacin,
	  clarithromycin, erythromycin, metronidazole,
	  norfloxacin, TMP-SMX
	certain anticonvulsants: carbamazepine,
	  ethosuximide, phenobarbital, phenytoin
	  primidone
	certain antifungals: fluconazole,
	  itraconazole, ketoconazole
	certain anti-ulcer drugs: cimetidine, omeprazole
	certain statins: fluvastatin, lovastatin
	  grapefruit juice
	other drugs: acetaminophen, cyclosporine,
	  dexamethasone, propafenone, rifabutin,
	  rifampin, zafirlukast
	other heart drugs: amiodarone, diltiazem,
	  quinine, verapamil

Beta-Blockers	
The drug below ...	**may interact with ...**
any beta-blocker	clonidine, digoxin, diltiazem, dipyridamole, disopyramide, prazosin, quinidine, theophylline, verapamil
atenolol	ampicillin
carvedilol	*anti-inflammatory medications* (e.g., ibuprofen, naproxen)
metoprolol	amiodarone, cimetidine, *anti-inflammatory medications* (e.g., ibuprofen, naproxen, propafenone)
propranolol	chlorpromazine, flecainide, fluoxetine, propoxyphene
metoprolol propranolol	carbamazepine, clomipramine, desipramine, fluoxetine, fluphenazone, haloperidol, paroxetine, propafenone, quinidine, phenobarbital, phenytoin, rifampin, ritonavir
bisoprolol timolol	sertraline, thioridazine

ACE Inhibitors	
The drug below ...	**may interact with ...**
any ACE inhibitor	allopurinol, aspirin, bumetanide, doxazosin, ethacrynic acid, furosemide, lithium, prazosin, terazosin

Cholesterol-Lowering Drugs	
The drug below . . .	**may interact with . . .**
bile acid resins	digoxin, warfarin, most other drugs
fibrates	glyburide, warfarin
certain statins	*certain antibiotics:* clarithromycin, erythromycin, metronidazole, norfloxacin *certain anticonvulsants:* carbamazepine, ethosuximide, phenobarbital, phenytoin *certain antidepressants:* fluoxetine, nefazodone, sertraline *certain antifungals:* fluconazole, itraconazole, ketoconazole *certain antivirals:* ritonavir, saquinavir *other cholesterol-lowering drugs:* cholestyramine, colestipol, niacin, gemfibrozil *other drugs:* cyclosporine, dexamethasone, primidone, rifabutin, rifampin, zafirlukast *other heart drugs:* amiodarone, diltiazem, quinine, verapamil, warfarin grapefruit juice

Blood Pressure–Lowering Drugs	
The drug below . . .	**may interact with . . .**
losartan	*certain antibiotics:* clarithromycin, erythromycin, metronidazole, norfloxacin, TMP/SMX *certain anticonvulsants:* carbamazepine, ethosuximide, phenobarbital, phenytoin, primidone *certain antidepressants:* fluoxetine, fluvoxamine, nefazodone, sertraline

The drug below . . .	may interact with . . .
	certain antifungals: fluconazole, itraconazole, ketoconazole *certain antivirals:* ritonavir, saquinavir *other drugs:* cimetidine, cyclosporine, dexamethasone, omeprazole, quinine, rifabutin, rifampin, zafirlukast *other heart drugs:* amiodarone, diltiazem, fluvastatin, verapamil grapefruit juice
certain calcium channel–blockers	amiodarone, atorvastatin, beta-blockers, carbamazepine, cimetidine, cyclosporine, digoxin, ethanol, grapefruit juice, itraconazole, nafcillin, omeprazole, ovastatin, phenytoin, quinidine, simvastatin
certain diuretics (also known as "water pills")	amikacin, certain anti-inflammatory medications (e.g., ibuprofen, naproxen), cholestyramine, colestipol, digoxin, ergotamine, gentamicin, mitotane, sildenafil, tobramycin

Other Heart Drugs	
The drug below . . .	**may interact with . . .**
digoxin	*certain anti-inflammatory medications* (e.g., ibuprofen, naproxen) *certain herbals:* e.g., buckthorn, cascara sagrada, senna, oleander, St. John's wort *other drugs:* charcoal, erythromycin, propafenone fluconazole, itraconazole, ketoconazole *other heart drugs:* amiodarone, any beta-blocker, diltiazem, propafenone, quinidine, spironolactone, verapamil
nitrates	sildenafil

Some Key Interactions to Watch Out For

NEVER COMBINE NITROGLYCERINE WITH VIAGRA OR CIALIS. It is very dangerous to take sildenafil (brand name: Viagra) or tadalafil (brand name: Cialis) while taking any nitrate-based heart medication, such as nitroglycerin tablets or isosorbide dinitrate (Isordil). The combined effect of these medications can drop your blood pressure to a level so low that it is life threatening.

BE CAUTIOUS WHEN TAKING MORE THAN ONE BLOOD THINNER AT A TIME. Aspirin, clopidogrel, and warfarin are a few of the many medications that fall under the category of blood thinners. Taking more than one of these at a time, even for specific medical reasons, may put you at a higher risk of bleeds—though sometimes the benefits may outweigh the risks. Taking one of these along with certain anti-inflammatory or pain medications, such as ibuprofen and naproxen (commonly used for arthritis), can also increase your risk of stomach bleeding in particular. Ask your doctor if your pain medication might interact with your blood thinner.

WATCH OUT FOR GRAPEFRUIT JUICE. Drinking grapefruit juice can have surprising effects on how your heart medications work. Grapefruit juice can increase the effect of the beta-blocker propranolol and can decrease the effect of statins (e.g., simvastatin, atorvastatin, lovastatin). To be safe, it may be best to avoid drinking grapefruit juice altogether.

BE AWARE OF MEDICATIONS THAT FIGHT INFECTION. While most are safe, certain antibiotics and antifungals commonly used to fight infection may have unwanted interactions with medications for your heart. See the previous charts for details.

Tests and Medical Procedures

Over the course of your heart disease treatment, your doctor will order any of several tests and procedures. Some measure and subsequently keep track of your risk factors. Others measure directly the status of your heart. Some of the procedures in this latter group involve surgery, and since every invasive procedure entails a degree of risk, it's important for you and your family to learn as much about the procedure as you can. In this regard, a number of studies suggest that patients do better when they are treated at hospitals where many of these procedures, such as angioplasty or coronary artery bypass surgery, are performed each year. Of course, the experience and skill of individual doctors can overcome this finding, but if you have a choice, you may choose to have such procedures done where the practitioners have the greatest experience.

Measuring and Tracking Risk Factors

In addition to checking your blood pressure regularly, your doctor may order any or all of the following tests or procedures.

Cholesterol and Triglycerides

ABOUT THE TEST: Measures of your blood cholesterol level can be done at any time, but the most accurate measures are taken after you have fasted for twelve hours or so. That is why the test is often done in the morning before you eat breakfast. A complete cholesterol and triglycerides test, also known as a "lipid panel," includes a measure of LDL (bad) cholesterol, HDL (good) cholesterol, total cholesterol, and triglycerides.

WHEN TO DO THE TEST: This test should be done every year or so if you do not have high "bad" cholesterol levels. For people being treated, the levels should be checked six weeks after starting a new cholesterol-lowering therapy and then every four to six months thereafter.

WHAT THE RESULTS MEAN: High LDL (bad) cholesterol, total cholesterol, and triglyceride levels and/or low HDL (good) cholesterol levels indicate that you have *dyslipidemia*—a condition that needs to be treated with cholesterol-lowering medication.

Glucose

ABOUT THE TEST: A measure of your blood glucose (sugar) can be done at any time, but the most meaningful measure for the diagnosis of diabetes is taken after you have not eaten for about twelve hours. Both fasting and non-fasting (random) glucose tests can be done by some patients in their own homes using a glucometer (glucose measuring device).

WHEN TO DO THE TEST: People with heart disease should have their fasting glucose measured at least every two years. People with diabetes need to have fasting and random glucose levels checked more frequently—up to a few times per day in some cases.

WHAT THE RESULTS MEAN: A fasting glucose level that is borderline high (between 110 and 126 mg/dL) should be monitored carefully. A fasting glucose level that is definitely high and that has been measured on at least two separate occasions means that you have diabetes and need to start diabetes therapies.

Hemoglobin A1c

ABOUT THE TEST: A measure of the hemoglobin A1c level in your blood indicates how much glucose (sugar) your blood cells have been exposed to on average over the last two to four months. This test level stays relatively constant over time, so it won't change as a result of a recent meal or medication just taken. Therefore, this is the best test for understanding how your glucose control has been over the longer term.

WHEN TO DO THE TEST: The test should be done every three months for people who have diabetes.

WHAT THE RESULTS MEAN: A high hemoglobin A1c level (7 percent or greater) means that your glucose levels have been on average higher than they should have been over the last few months. This means that your current strategy for controlling your glucose levels needs to be adjusted.

Blood Chemistry

ABOUT THE TEST: Blood levels of key minerals and proteins are measured to monitor how certain blood pressure–lowering medications may be affecting the kidneys. The elements measured can include: sodium, potassium, chloride, bicarbonate, and more specific measures of kidney function called urea nitrogen and creatinine. These measures are also done to help monitor hypertension or heart failure.

WHEN TO DO THE TEST: These measures are checked before starting blood pressure–lowering medication and then periodically afterward. They may be done more frequently in people who have heart failure or who are being treated with diuretics. High potassium levels may be a particular problem for patients on ACE inhibitors or aldosterone antagonists.

WHAT THE RESULTS MEAN: Abnormal levels of the elements measured in blood chemistry can be a sign of wear on the kidneys as a result of high blood pressure, certain blood pressure medications, or heart failure.

Measuring and Tracking the Status of Your Heart Disease

You and your doctor will want to know whether your heart disease has gotten worse, stayed the same, or gotten better. The tests and procedures below are those that are most commonly used. You don't need to have all of these tests done for your doctor to understand and effectively monitor the status of your heart disease.

Electrocardiography

ABOUT THE TEST: Also known as an EKG or ECG, this is a painless and noninvasive test used to record the pattern of electrical currents generated by the heart. Wires are placed across your chest and on each of your limbs to pick up the electrical activity. All you need to do is lie flat for a few minutes.

WHEN TO DO THE TEST: An ECG test is often done when there is a change in the symptoms or signs of heart disease—and sometimes just for monitoring purposes. An ECG is also often done if there is a suspicion that the heart is beating at an unusual rate or rhythm.

WHAT THE RESULTS MEAN: Different patterns from an ECG tracing can show that a part of the heart is not getting enough blood supply, that there has been a heart attack in the past, or that the heart rate or rhythm has unusual features. However, an ECG tracing can also appear normal in people who have heart disease—which is why other diagnostic tests are often needed.

Holter Monitoring

ABOUT THE TEST: Also called "ambulatory ECG," this test is like an ECG test, only instead of getting a heart tracing over a few minutes, a similar monitoring device is worn by the patient for at least twenty-four hours while performing daily activities and a continuous heart tracing is recorded over this period of time. This test is also called a "Holter monitor," named for the person who developed it.

WHEN TO DO THE TEST: A Holter test is often done if a patient has fainted or has unexplained episodes of feeling light-headed, dizzy, or weak, or of palpitations. The test can show if these symptoms are related to periods of abnormal heart rate or rhythm over the course of a day.

WHAT THE RESULTS MEAN: The results can indicate conditions that need further evaluation or treatment based on the heart's electrical activity.

Exercise Stress Test

ABOUT THE TEST: This is a noninvasive test that involves wearing wires connected to a machine that monitors heartbeat, blood pressure, and ECG tracing while the patient performs various levels of exercise on a treadmill or stationary bicycle.

WHEN TO DO THE TEST: An exercise stress test is done to help make the diagnosis of heart disease for people who experience chest pain or difficulty breathing. For people who already have heart disease, the test can help determine how serious the condition is.

WHAT THE RESULTS MEAN: This test can help determine whether your heart is receiving an adequate blood flow during exertion. Doctors evaluate how long you can exercise, what happens to your heart rate and blood pressure during exertion, whether you develop any symptoms, whether your electrocardiogram shows important changes, and how your heart rate recovers after you finish. This test helps the doctor know whether your risk of future heart disease is high and whether additional tests might be useful to you. Sometimes, particularly for people with difficult-to-interpret electrocardiograms, pictures of the heart are taken (see Nuclear Scan, on the following page).

Echocardiography

ABOUT THE TEST: This is a painless, noninvasive but effective way to see what your heart looks like and how it is working. Some lubricant jelly is placed on your chest and then a special ultrasound probe is rolled along the jelly to take both moving and snapshot pictures of your heart as you lie still. Another type of ultrasound test that is done less commonly involves swallowing a smaller ultrasound probe in order to obtain better pictures of your heart. Patients usually receive medication to relax them for this test. It is called a transesophageal echocardiogram (TEE) and is much less frequently required. The advantage of TEE is that the pictures are much better, and it is only required when the other ultrasound test does not provide good enough pictures for what the doctor is trying to see.

WHEN TO DO THE TEST: Echocardiography is often done when there is a change in the symptoms or signs of heart disease. An echocardiogram can be done to assess an enlarged heart, abnormal sounds (such as murmurs), unexplained chest pain, difficulty breathing, palpitations, and stroke (which can be caused by blood clots from the heart). An echocardiogram can also be combined with an exercise test to evaluate blood flow to the heart.

WHAT THE RESULTS MEAN: The results of an echocardiogram can help confirm the diagnosis of heart disease, measure the ability of the heart to do its job of pumping blood to the rest of the body, and indicate whether there are any abnormalities of the heart valves or heart walls.

Nuclear Scan

ABOUT THE TEST: During this test, a small amount of radio-active substance (such as thallium or technium) is injected into your bloodstream. Although it is radioactive, the dose is so small that it is not considered dangerous, even for people who have this test many times over their lifetime. As the substance travels to the arteries that supply blood to your heart muscle, a camera scans the amount of the radioactive substance reaching different parts of the heart muscle while you exercise. The distribution of the substance can tell the doctors about the blood flow to your heart. If it is not possible for you to exercise, another substance is injected to simulate exercise-like stress on the heart while the scan is being done. The stress medication may cause you to have some discomfort (e.g., headache, nausea, chest pain, shortness of breath) for a few minutes, but these symptoms should not last long. After the exercise or stress-medication part of the test is done, you will usually be asked to rest for about four hours before another scan is done. The two scans are then compared to identify the size and location of poor blood supply or damage to your heart muscle.

WHEN TO DO THE TEST: A nuclear scan is similar to an exercise stress test but provides more information about blood flow through the coronary arteries. Your doctor may order a nuclear scan if you have worsening symptoms and more information is needed about the condition of your heart—and particularly when the electrocardiogram has certain patterns that are difficult to interpret in an exercise test.

WHAT THE RESULTS MEAN: A nuclear scan can show if a part of your heart that is deprived of blood supply during exercise can recover after rest—this result would suggest narrowed arteries. If an area of the heart does not get any blood supply during exercise and does not recover after rest, this area is likely to have scar tissue left over from a previous heart attack.

Electron-Beam Computerized Tomography

ABOUT THE TEST: Also known as EBCT or a CT artery scan, this test involves taking pictures of the arteries that supply the heart to determine whether there are any areas of blood vessel hardening and narrowing. Arteries that are hardened and narrowed by heart disease will have calcium deposits in the vessel walls, and this is what the computerized tomography (CT) scan picks up. All the patient has to do is lie still in the CT scanner while it takes high-resolution pictures of the heart. Since this test is relatively new, the American Heart Association/American College of Cardiology are waiting for more studies of its use before fully recommending this test to help diagnose heart disease.

WHEN TO DO THE TEST: Although not yet widely used, this test is done to help diagnose heart disease, especially if the patient does not yet have symptoms. Because the test is simple to perform, it may be used more in the future as a way to screen for narrowed or blocked major arteries of the heart in people who have a high risk for heart disease.

WHAT THE RESULTS MEAN: Pictures taken during this test will show whether one or more of the major arteries of the heart is hardened or narrowed by heart disease.

Electrophysiology Test

ABOUT THE TEST: Heart disease makes some people's hearts more prone to beating with an irregular rhythm or rate (arrhythmia). Also known as an EP study or EP testing, electrophysiology testing is used to help diagnose this condition, especially if it is not obvious from other testing. The test involves threading a small wire into the heart in the same way as is done during a cardiac catheterization. Once the tip of the wire is in the heart, it can then be used to directly stimulate and record electrical signals made by the heart and to perform tests from various locations inside the heart. If needed, the area causing the irregularity can be targeted for special treatment or a pacemaker can be placed in the heart at the time of the test.

WHEN TO DO THE TEST: This test is done when it is suspected that a person's heart may be beating with a dangerous rhythm. Sometimes the clue is fainting episodes or episodes of rapid or slow heart rates (which can be associated with a fluttering feeling inside one's chest).

WHAT THE RESULTS MEAN: The results of the test indicate whether a person's heart is prone to beating irregularly, and if so, what kind of an irregularity (arrhythmia) it is. This helps determine how it should be treated.

Cardiac Catheterization

ABOUT THE TEST: This test and procedure is also known as a "coronary angiogram." A small amount of numbing medication is placed in your groin or arm and a thin, flexible tube (catheter) is inserted at that site and then guided painlessly up to the coronary arteries (the blood vessels that supply blood to your heart muscle). A dye is then injected through the tube and, as the dye flows into and through the coronary arteries, X-ray video pictures are taken. Many people feel a brief warm or hot sensation in their chest from the dye.

WHEN TO DO THE TEST: This procedure is done if a patient experiences new or worsening symptoms, suggesting that there is not enough blood and oxygen reaching the heart muscle. The catheterization may also be done after a positive exercise or nuclear test.

WHAT THE RESULTS MEAN: Pictures taken during this procedure will show whether one or more of the major arteries supplying the heart muscle with blood is narrowed or blocked. If a major artery is found to be narrowed, your doctor may decide that angioplasty—with or without stenting—should be done at that moment to widen the area of narrowing. Certain findings may suggest the need for surgery.

Percutaneous Coronary Interventions

ABOUT THE PROCEDURE: These interventions, also known as PCI, include angioplasty and stenting and are often performed in the same way as a cardiac catheterization. During *angioplasty*, a doctor threads a small deflated balloon through the catheter to the site of coronary artery narrowing. The balloon is then inflated with air, causing the plaque that is narrowing the vessel to be flattened against the vessel wall and allowing more room for blood to flow through. As the balloon is inflated, you may feel some angina-like discomfort which you should tell your doctor about at that time. The balloon is then deflated. *Stenting* is often done next. A coronary stent is a special expandable mesh tube that is placed over the deflated balloon. The balloon is then inflated one more time so that the stent expands and is fitted into the artery wall against the flattened plaque. The balloon is then deflated and removed while the stent is left in place to keep the artery propped open. Some new types of stents, called "drug-eluting stents," slowly release a medication that helps to keep an artery from reclosing after the stent is put in place.

WHEN TO DO THE PROCEDURE: These interventions can be done during a cardiac catheterization when the pictures show an area of vessel narrowing. Angioplasty with or without stenting can also be done if you are having a heart attack, to rapidly restore blood flow to the heart.

WHAT IS THE RESULT? When used during a heart attack, these interventions can return blood flow to an area of the heart that might otherwise become damaged and scarred. In non–heart attack situations, angioplasty can improve angina and related symptoms of heart disease. Stenting lowers the risk that the area of the coronary artery will reclose. How well angioplasty and stenting work to prevent future heart problems or prolong life is still being studied. It seems that they are most useful for improving quality of life.

Coronary Artery Bypass Grafting Surgery

ABOUT THE PROCEDURE: Also known as CABG (pronounced "cabbage") or "bypass surgery," this is a major operation done under general anesthesia, and it usually lasts anywhere from two to six hours. During the operation, a piece of vein from your leg or an artery from your chest is used to reroute or bypass blood around a blocked segment of artery. It may be done by opening the chest, though occasionally only a small incision is made in the chest (in what is called "minimally invasive surgery").

WHEN TO DO THE PROCEDURE: If angioplasty is unsuccessful or if cardiac catheterization shows that the artery blockage is too complex for angioplasty, or if you have severe blockages in many major arteries, your doctor may recommend bypass surgery. Bypass surgery is also recommended instead of angioplasty for many people with diabetes.

WHAT IS THE RESULT? Bypass surgery is not a cure for heart disease. As with angioplasty, bypass surgery works to improve heart disease symptoms and potentially reduce your risk of future heart problems. It is useful to know if this surgery is being recommended to you to improve the quality of your life or to increase the length of your life. Only certain types of patients are thought to derive survival benefit from CABG; for most people the surgery is primarily to improve the quality of their life.

National Research-Based Organizations

American Diabetes Association (ADA)
http://www.diabetes.org

American Heart Association (AHA)
http://www.americanheart.org

National Institutes of Health (NIH)
http://www.nih.gov

National Heart, Lung, and Blood Institute (NHLBI)
http://www.nhlbi.nih.gov

Patient-Oriented Information About Heart Disease

Heartinfo.org
http://www.heartinfo.org

My Heart Watch (sponsored by AHA)
http://www.myheartwatch.org

Virtual Office of the Surgeon General
http://www.surgeongeneral.gov

WebMD
http://my.webmd.com/condition_center/cvd

Support for Patients and Families

Mended Hearts
http://www.mendedhearts.org

About Quitting Smoking

Surgeon General's Website
http://www.surgeongeneral.gov/tobacco

For a free copy of the consumer brochure "You Can Quit Smoking," call any of the numbers below:

- Agency for Healthcare Research and Quality (AHRQ): 1-800-358-9295

- Centers for Disease Control and Prevention (CDC): 1-800-CDC-1311

- National Cancer Institute (NCI): 1-800-4-CANCER

ACC American College of Cardiology, the national professional organization for cardiologists.

ACE inhibitors Also known as "angiotensin-converting enzyme" inhibitors. These medications are used to lower risk of future heart problems in people with heart disease. These medications can also be used to lower blood pressure and to treat people with heart failure. Generic names for ACE inhibitors include: ramipril, captopril, enalapril, lisinopril, etc.

AHA American Heart Association, the national organization that sponsors research and public health programs concerning heart disease.

angina Typically chest pain or chest tightness (though it can be manifest as other symptoms) that is caused by heart disease. Angina usually occurs when a person with heart disease is under physical or other stress. When angina occurs at rest, the patient should immediately let his or her doctor know, because it may be a signal of an impending heart attack.

angioplasty A procedure in which a small balloon is inflated at the site of a narrowed coronary artery to open it up. This is often followed by putting a wire mesh stent at the site to help decrease the chance that the artery will reclose.

angiotensin II receptor blockers Medications that are thought to have a similar effect as ACE inhibitors but that work by a slightly different mechanism. Like ACE inhibitors, they are known to be useful for lowering blood pressure.

anticoagulant drugs   Medications that reduce the chance that clots will form in the bloodstream. Examples include heparin and warfain.

antioxidants   Although oxygen is necessary for the body, it can be broken down to form "free radicals," which are particles that can cause damage to cells. It is thought that having too many free radicals can lead to cancer, heart disease, or stroke. Antioxidants are molecules that "turn off" free radicals. Antioxidants are found in vitamins, fruits, and vegetables.

arrhythmia   A condition in which the heartbeat has an abnormal rate or rhythm.

atherosclerosis   The process of hardening of the arteries that can lead to heart disease. See "plaque."

beta-blockers   Medications used to reduce blood pressure, treat angina and heart failure, and generally help protect a heart affected by heart disease from further problems.

bypass surgery   See "coronary artery bypass grafting."

CABG   See "coronary artery bypass grafting."

CAD   See "coronary artery disease."

calcium channel–blockers   Medications used to help lower blood pressure, to treat angina, and in some cases to help control irregular heart rates and rhythms.

calorie   A measure of the amount of energy a person gets from eating a certain amount of food. Fats have more than twice the amount of calories per gram than carbohydrates or protein.

cardiac catheterization   A special procedure done to take a close look at a person's coronary arteries. This procedure is performed in a special laboratory by a cardiologist. A thin flexible tube (catheter) is threaded through your blood vessels to reach the coronary arteries and dye is then pushed through the tube so that pictures of the flow of the dye can be taken.

cardiovascular disease   Disease that affects the heart or the system of blood vessels that supplies the body with oxygen (the arterial vascular system of the body).

CDC   Centers for Disease Control and Prevention, an agency of the U.S. Department of Health and Human Services.

coronary arteries   The blood vessels that supply the heart muscle with oxygen. In heart disease, these arteries narrow, harden, or get blocked.

coronary artery bypass grafting   Also known as CABG (pronounced "cabbage") surgery. This is an operation in which one or more blood vessels (usually taken from a patient's leg or chest) are used to bypass a narrowed artery in the heart and in this way improve the heart's blood supply.

coronary artery disease   Heart disease caused by narrowing of the blood vessels that feed the heart muscle.

diastolic blood pressure   The pressure in the arteries when the heart relaxes between beats. This pressure is reflected in the bottom number in a blood pressure reading.

diuretics   Also known as "water pills," these medications are used to lower blood pressure or treat heart failure.

echocardiogram   A diagnostic test that uses ultrasound waves to take pictures of the heart as it beats. An echocardiogram provides information about the structure and function of the different parts of the heart.

ejection fraction   The percentage of blood in the heart at any given moment that leaves the largest chamber of the heart with each heartbeat. The ejection fraction is normally between 50 and 65 percent in a healthy person.

electrocardiogram   Also known as an ECG or EKG, this is a record of electrical activity of the heart. The ECG is used to determine if there are any irregularities of heart rate or rhythm or if any part of the heart is not getting enough blood flow or has been damaged in the past.

glucose   This is the most basic form of sugar. "Glucose level" usually refers to the level of sugar in the bloodstream. This is important to monitor in people with diagnosed or suspected diabetes.

HDL cholesterol   The "good" type of cholesterol. People with heart disease should aim to have their HDL cholesterol level above 40 mg/dL.

heart failure   A condition in which the heart is weakened and cannot pump as much blood as it needs to with each beat.

Heart failure can often be the result of long-standing high blood pressure and/or heart disease.

Holter monitor A portable ECG machine that is worn, usually for 24 hours, to continuously monitor the heart's electrical activity while a person performs daily activities.

hormone-replacement therapy Female hormone medications commonly prescribed to women who experience severe symptoms of menopause or who are at high risk of osteoporosis-related problems after menopause.

HRT See "hormone-replacement therapy."

hypercholesterolemia Condition of having high cholesterol.

hyperglycemia Condition of having high blood glucose (sugar).

hyperlipidemia Condition of having high cholesterol.

hypertension Condition of having high blood pressure.

ischemic The medical term that describes a state in which there is not enough blood and oxygen reaching a particular part of the body. During a heart attack, a part of the heart muscle becomes ischemic.

LDL cholesterol The "bad" type of cholesterol. People with heart disease should aim to have their LDL cholesterol level below 100 mg/dL.

n-omega 3 fatty acids The type of fatty acids that are found in fatty fish as well as certain vegetable products. Regular consumption of these fatty acids has been linked to improved heart health.

NIH National Institutes of Health, the federal government organization in charge of medical research.

nitroglycerin A medication in tablet or spray form that is used to relieve angina (chest pain) as soon as it happens.

myocardial infarction Medical term for heart attack.

myocardial ischemia Condition in which the heart muscle is not getting enough blood and oxygen. This condition may be reversed without leaving permanent damage to the heart muscle—or it can lead to a full heart attack.

myocardium The medical term for the heart muscle.

PCI See "percutaneous coronary intervention."

percutaneous coronary intervention   A procedure that takes place during cardiac catheterization. The procedure is often angioplasty (inflation of a balloon to widen a narrowed artery) followed by stenting (permanent placement of a piece of wire mesh tube in a previously narrowed coronary artery to keep it wide open).

plaque   A buildup of cholesterol-based substances, smooth muscle cells, proteins, and calcium in the wall of an artery. As plaques grow larger over time, they narrow the opening of the artery to the point where blood cannot flow through as easily.

polyunsaturated fat   The kind of fat found in safflower, sunflower, and corn oils. Consuming polyunsaturated fat instead of saturated fat can help lower your LDL cholesterol levels.

presyncope   Condition in which you feel light-headed, as if you are about to faint, because there is reduced blood flow getting to the brain.

randomized controlled trial   The "gold standard" of research studies that investigate the effect of treatments. A therapy is tested out by taking a large sample of study subjects and randomly giving one portion of the subjects the therapy and another portion of the subjects a placebo. Afterward, researchers can determine how the therapy works in comparison to placebo.

saturated fat   The kind of fat that comes from animals and certain oils, such as palm oil and coconut oil. Consuming saturated fats increases blood cholesterol levels.

stable angina   The most common type of angina, this is chest pain caused by heart disease that has a predictable pattern and is not getting worse. It typically comes on with exertion and is relieved by rest or a small dose of nitroglycerin (tablets or spray). See "angina."

stent   A piece of wire mesh tubing made out of high-quality stainless steel. A stent is commonly placed at the site of coronary artery narrowing after angioplasty. See "angioplasty."

syncope   Condition in which you temporarily lose consciousness (or faint) because there is not enough blood flow getting to the brain.

systolic blood pressure   The pressure felt by the arteries during each squeezing action of the heart, between periods of relaxation. The systolic blood pressure is reflected in the top number that is part of the blood pressure reading.

thrombus   The medical term for blood clot.

triglycerides   A type of fat that can build up in the blood to cause atherosclerosis. Triglycerides contribute to the total cholesterol count in the blood.

unstable angina   Angina (chest pain) that comes on in an unpredictable manner, that is getting worse, or that is not easily relieved by rest or nitroglycerin. People who experience unstable angina should call or see a doctor right away.

REFERENCES

Chapter 1. Understanding Heart Disease

Magnus, P., and R. Beaglehole. The real contribution of the major risk factors to the coronary epidemics: time to end the "only-50%" myth. *Archives of Internal Medicine*, 2001, Vol. 161, Iss. 22, 2657–2660.

Murray, C. J., et al. Effectiveness and costs of interventions to lower systolic blood pressure and cholesterol: a global and regional analysis on reduction of cardiovascular-disease risk. *Lancet*, 2003, Vol. 361, Iss. 9359, 717–725.

Ornato, J. P., and M. M. Hand. Warning signs of a heart attack. *Circulation*, 2001, Vol. 104, Iss. 11, 1212–1213.

Chapter 2. Seven Key Strategies for Taking Charge of Heart Disease

Smith, S. C., Jr., et al. AHA/ACC scientific statement: AHA/ACC guidelines for preventing heart attack and death in patients with atherosclerotic cardiovascular disease: 2001 update: a statement for healthcare professionals from the American Heart Association and the American College of Cardiology. *Circulation*, 2001, Vol. 104, Iss. 13, 1577–1579.

Strategy #1: Take Charge of Your Blood Pressure

Benson, H., J. B. Kotch, and K. D. Crassweller. Stress and hypertension: interrelations and management. *Cardiovascular Clinics*, 1978, Vol. 9, Iss. 1, 113–124.

Dahlof, B., et al. Cardiovascular morbidity and mortality in the Losartan Intervention For Endpoint Reduction in Hypertension study (LIFE): a randomised trial against atenolol. *Lancet*, 2002, Vol. 359, Iss. 9311, 995–1003.

Douglas, J. G., et al. Management of high blood pressure in African Americans: consensus statement of the Hypertension in African Americans Working Group of the International Society on Hypertension in Blacks. *Archives of Internal Medicine*, 2003, Vol. 163, Iss. 5, 525–541.

Furberg, C. D., et al. Clinical implications of recent findings from the Antihypertensive and Lipid-Lowering Treatment to Prevent Heart Attack Trial (ALLHAT) and other studies of hypertension. *Annals of Internal Medicine*, 2001, Vol. 135, Iss. 12, 1074–1078.

Hyman, D. J., and V. N. Pavlik. Characteristics of patients with uncontrolled hypertension in the United States. *New England Journal of Medicine*, 2001, Vol. 345, Iss. 7, 479–486.

Jones, D. W., et al. Measuring blood pressure accurately: new and persistent challenges. *Journal of the American Medical Association*, 2003, Vol. 289, Iss. 8, 1027–1030.

Lindholm, L. H., et al. Cardiovascular morbidity and mortality in patients with diabetes in the Losartan Intervention For Endpoint Reduction in Hypertension study (LIFE): a randomised trial against atenolol. *Lancet*, 2002, Vol. 359, Iss. 9311, 1004–1010.

Major outcomes in high-risk hypertensive patients randomized to angiotensin-converting enzyme inhibitor or calcium channel blocker vs diuretic: The Antihypertensive and Lipid-Lowering Treatment to Prevent Heart Attack Trial (ALLHAT). The ALLHAT Officers and Coordinators for the ALLHAT Collaborative Research Group. *Journal of the American Medical Association*, 2002, Vol. 288, Iss. 23, 2981–2997.

Moser, M. White-coat hypertension—to treat or not to treat: a clinical dilemma. *Archives of Internal Medicine*, 2001, Vol. 161, Iss. 22, 2655–2656.

Neal, B., S. MacMahon, and N. Chapman. Effects of ACE inhibitors, calcium antagonists, and other blood-pressure-lowering drugs: results of prospectively designed overviews of randomised trials. Blood Pressure Lowering Treatment Trialists' Collaboration. *Lancet*, 2000, Vol. 356, Iss. 9246, 1955–1964.

The seventh report of the Joint National Committee on Prevention, Detection, Evaluation, and Treatment of High Blood Pressure. National Institutes of Health, National Heart, Lung, and Blood Institute, 2003.

Shekelle, P. G., et al. Efficacy and safety of ephedra and ephedrine for weight loss and athletic performance: a meta-analysis. *Journal of the American Medical Association*, 2003, Vol. 289, Iss. 12, 1537–1545.

The sixth report of the Joint National Committee on Prevention, Detection, Evaluation, and Treatment of High Blood Pressure. National Institutes of Health, National Heart, Lung, and Blood Institute, 1997.

Staessen, J. A., et al. Risks of untreated and treated isolated systolic hypertension in the elderly: meta-analysis of outcome trials. *Lancet*, 2000, Vol. 355, Iss. 9207, 865–872.

Vasan, R. S., et al. Residual lifetime risk for developing hypertension in middle-aged women and men: The Framingham Heart Study. *Journal of the American Medical Association*, 2002, Vol. 287, Iss. 8, 1003–1010.

Vollmer, W. M., et al. Effects of diet and sodium intake on blood pressure: subgroup analysis of the DASH-sodium trial. *Annals of Internal Medicine*, 2001, Vol. 135, Iss. 12, 1019–1028.

Wing, L. M., et al. A comparison of outcomes with angiotensin-converting-enzyme inhibitors and diuretics for hypertension in the elderly. *New England Journal of Medicine*, 2003, Vol. 348, Iss. 7, 583–592.

Strategy #2: Take Charge of Your Cholesterol

Cannon, C. P., et al. Intensive versus moderate lipid lowering with statins after acute coronary syndromes. *New England Journal of Medicine*, 2004, Vol. 350, Iss. 15, 1494–1504.

Chong, P. H., J. D. Seeger, and C. Franklin. Clinically relevant differences between the statins: implications for therapeutic selection. *American Journal of Medicine*, 2001, Vol. 111, Iss. 5, 390–400.

Davidson, M. H. Treatment of the elderly with 3-hydroxy-3-methylglutaryl coenzyme A reductase inhibitors: focus on drug interactions. *Journal of Cardiovascular Pharmacology and Therapeutics*, 2001, Vol. 6, Iss. 3, 219–229.

Dresser, G. K., and D. G. Bailey. A basic conceptual and practical overview of interactions with highly prescribed drugs. *Canadian Journal of Clinical Pharmacology*, 2002, Vol. 9, Iss. 4, 191–198.

Executive summary of the third report of the National Cholesterol Education Program (NCEP) Expert Panel on Detection, Evaluation, and Treatment of High Blood Cholesterol in Adults (Adult Treatment Panel III). *Journal of the American Medical Association*, 2001, Vol. 285, Iss. 2486–2497.

Feely, J. The therapeutic gap—compliance with medication and guidelines. *Atherosclerosis*, 1999, Vol. 147, Suppl. 1, S31–S37.

Ford, E. S., et al. Serum total cholesterol concentrations and awareness, treatment, and control of hypercholesterolemia among US adults: findings from the National Health and Nutrition Examination Survey, 1999 to 2000. *Circulation*, 2003, Vol. 107, Iss. 17, 2185–2189.

Ginsberg, H. N., et al. Effects of reducing dietary saturated fatty acids on plasma lipids and lipoproteins in healthy subjects: the DELTA Study, protocol 1. *Arteriosclerosis, Thrombosis and Vascular Biology*, 1998, Vol. 18, Iss. 3, 441–449.

Heart disease: from cause to cure. *New York Times* special supplement, February 23, 2003, 5.

Igel, M., T. Sudhop, and K. von Bergmann. Metabolism and drug interactions of 3-hydroxy-3-methylglutaryl coenzyme A-reductase inhibitors (statins). *European Journal of Clinical Pharmacology*, 2001, Vol. 57, Iss. 5, 357–364.

Jula, A., et al. Effects of diet and simvastatin on serum lipids, insulin, and antioxidants in hypercholesterolemic men: a randomized controlled trial. *Journal of the American Medical Association*, 2002, Vol. 287, Iss. 5, 598–605.

Kantola, T., K. T. Kivisto, and P. J. Neuvonen. Grapefruit juice greatly increases serum concentrations of lovastatin and lovastatin acid. *Clinical Pharmacology and Therapeutics*, 1998, Vol. 63, Iss. 4, 397–402.

Kivipelto, M., et al. Apolipoprotein E epsilon4 allele, elevated midlife total cholesterol level, and high midlife systolic blood pressure are independent risk factors for late-life Alzheimer disease. *Annals of Internal Medicine*, 2002, Vol. 137, Iss. 3, 149–155.

Kraus, W. E., et al. Effects of the amount and intensity of exercise on plasma lipoproteins. *New England Journal of Medicine*, 2002, Vol. 347, Iss. 19, 1483–1492.

Lewis, S. J., et al. Effect of pravastatin on cardiovascular events in women after myocardial infarction: the cholesterol and recurrent events (CARE) trial. *Journal of the American College of Cardiology*, 1998, Vol. 32, Iss. 1, 140–146.

Lichtenstein, A. H., et al. Effects of different forms of dietary hydrogenated fats on serum lipoprotein cholesterol levels. *New England Journal of Medicine*, 1999, Vol. 340, Iss. 25, 1933–1940.

Lilja, J. J., K. T. Kivisto, and P. J. Neuvonen. Grapefruit juice increases serum concentrations of atorvastatin and has no effect on pravastatin. *Clinical Pharmacology and Therapeutics*, 1999, Vol. 66, Iss. 2, 118–127.

MRC/BHF Heart Protection Study of cholesterol lowering with simvastatin in 20,536 high-risk individuals: a randomised placebo-controlled trial. Heart Protection Study Collaborative Group. *Lancet*, 2002, Vol. 360, Iss. 9326, 7–22.

Pasternak, R. C., et al. ACC/AHA/NHLBI clinical advisory on the use and safety of statins. *Journal of the American College of Cardiology*, 2002, Vol. 40, Iss. 3, 567–572.

Phillips, P. S., et al. Statin-associated myopathy with normal creatine kinase levels. *Annals of Internal Medicine*, 2002, Vol. 137, Iss. 7, 581–585.

Prevention of cardiovascular events and death with pravastatin in patients with coronary heart disease and a broad range of initial cholesterol levels. The Long-Term Intervention with Pravastatin in Ischaemic Disease (LIPID) Study Group. *New England Journal of Medicine*, 1998, Vol. 339, Iss. 19, 1349–1357.

Randomised trial of cholesterol lowering in 4,444 patients with coronary heart disease: the Scandinavian Simvastatin Survival Study (4S). Scandinavian Simvastatin Survival Study Group. *Lancet*, 1994, Vol. 344, Iss. 8934, 1383–1389.

Rubins, H. B., et al. Gemfibrozil for the secondary prevention of coronary heart disease in men with low levels of high-density lipoprotein cholesterol. Veterans Affairs High-Density Lipoprotein Cholesterol Intervention Trial Study Group. *New England Journal of Medicine*, 1999, Vol. 341, Iss. 6, 410–418.

Smith, C. C., et al. Screening for statin-related toxicity: the yield of transaminase and creatine kinase measurements in a primary care setting. *Archives of Internal Medicine*, 2003, Vol. 163, Iss. 6, 688–692.

Sterzer, P., et al. Pravastatin improves cerebral vasomotor reactivity in patients with subcortical small-vessel disease. *Stroke*, 2001, Vol. 32, Iss. 12, 2817–2820.

Velasco, J. A. After 4S, CARE and LIPID—is evidence-based medicine being practised? *Atherosclerosis*, 1999, Vol. 147, Suppl. 1, S39–S44.

Virmani, R., et al. Coronary artery atherosclerosis revisited in Korean war combat casualties. *Archives of Pathology and Laboratory Medicine*, 1987, Vol. 111, Iss. 10, 972–976.

Walden, C. E., et al. Lipoprotein lipid response to the National Cholesterol Education Program step II diet by hypercholesterolemic and combined hyperlipidemic women and men. *Arteriosclerosis, Thrombosis and Vascular Biology*, 1997, Vol. 17, Iss. 2, 375–382.

Strategy #3: Take Charge of Your Fitness

Ades, P. A. Cardiac rehabilitation and secondary prevention of coronary heart disease. *New England Journal of Medicine*, 2001, Vol. 345, Iss. 12, 892–902.

Ades, P. A., and C. E. Coello. Effects of exercise and cardiac rehabilitation on cardiovascular outcomes. *Medical Clinics of North America*, 2000, Vol. 84, Iss. 1, 251–265, x-xi.

Albert, C. M., et al. Triggering of sudden death from cardiac causes by vigorous exertion. *New England Journal of Medicine*, 2000, Vol. 343, Iss. 19, 1355–1361.

Brassington, G. S., et al. Intervention-related cognitive versus social mediators of exercise adherence in the elderly. *American Journal of Preventive Medicine*, 2002, Vol. 23, Suppl. 1, 80–86.

Brechue, W. F., and M. L. Pollock. Exercise training for coronary artery disease in the elderly. *Clinics in Geriatric Medicine*, 1996, Vol. 12, Iss. 1, 207–229.

Brochu, M., et al. Modest effects of exercise training alone on coronary risk factors and body composition in coronary patients. *Journal of Cardiopulmonary Rehabilitation*, 2000, Vol. 20, Iss. 3, 180–188.

Cox, K. L., et al. Controlled comparison of retention and adherence in home- vs center-initiated exercise interventions in women ages 40–65 years: The S.W.E.A.T. Study (Sedentary Women Exercise Adherence Trial). *Preventive Medicine*, 2003, Vol. 36, Iss. 1, 17–29.

Despres, J. P., and B. Lamarche. Low-intensity endurance exercise training, plasma lipoproteins and the risk of coronary heart disease. *Journal of Internal Medicine*, 1994, Vol. 236, Iss. 1, 7–22.

Duncan, K. A., and B. Pozehl. Staying on course: the effects of an adherence facilitation intervention on home exercise participation. *Progress in Cardiovascular Nursing*, 2002, Vol. 17, Iss. 2, 59–65, 71.

Dunn, A. L., et al. Comparison of lifestyle and structured interventions to increase physical activity and cardiorespiratory fitness: a randomized trial. *Journal of the American Medical Association*, 1999, Vol. 281, Iss. 4, 327–334.

Eaton, C. B. Relation of physical activity and cardiovascular fitness to coronary heart disease, Part II: cardiovascular fitness and the safety and efficacy of physical activity prescription. *Journal of the American Board of Family Practice*, 1992, Vol. 5, Iss. 2, 157–165.

Fonarow, G. C., et al. Improved treatment of coronary heart disease by implementation of a Cardiac Hospitalization Atherosclerosis Management Program (CHAMP). *American Journal of Cardiology*, 2001, Vol. 87, Iss. 7, 819–822.

Gordon, N. F., and C. B. Scott. The role of exercise in the primary and secondary prevention of coronary artery disease. *Clinics in Sports Medicine*, 1991, Vol. 10, Iss. 1, 87–103.

Hakim, A. A., et al. Effects of walking on mortality among non-smoking retired men. *New England Journal of Medicine*, 1998, Vol. 338, Iss. 2, 94–99.

Hambrecht, R., et al. Various intensities of leisure time physical activity in patients with coronary artery disease: effects on cardiorespiratory fitness and progression of coronary atherosclerotic lesions. *Journal of the American College of Cardiology*, 1993, Vol. 22, Iss. 2, 468–477.

Hartley, L. H. The role of exercise in the primary and secondary prevention of atherosclerotic coronary artery disease. *Cardiovascular Clinics*, 1985, Vol. 15, Iss. 2, 1–8.

Houston, T. K., et al. Sports ability in young men and the incidence of cardiovascular disease. *American Journal of Medicine*, 2002, Vol. 112, Iss. 9, 689–695.

Iellamo, F., et al. Effects of a residential exercise training on baroreflex sensitivity and heart rate variability in patients with coronary artery disease: a randomized, controlled study. *Circulation*, 2000, Vol. 102, Iss. 21, 2588–2592.

Jacobs, D. R., Jr., and K. H. Schmitz. Tennis, anyone? On the value of sustainable, vigorous physical activity and long-term studies. *American Journal of Medicine*, 2002, Vol. 112, Iss. 9, 733–734.

Jolliffe, J. A., et al. Exercise-based rehabilitation for coronary heart disease. *Cochrane Database System Review*, 2000, Vol. 4, CD001800.

Kujala, U. M., et al. Relationship of leisure-time physical activity and mortality: the Finnish twin cohort. *Journal of the American Medical Association*, 1998, Vol. 279, Iss. 6, 440–444.

Lakka, T. A., et al. Relation of leisure-time physical activity and cardiorespiratory fitness to the risk of acute myocardial infarction. *New England Journal of Medicine*, 1994, Vol. 330, Iss. 22, 1549–1554.

Lavie, C. J., and R. V. Milani. Effects of cardiac rehabilitation and exercise training on exercise capacity, coronary risk factors, behavioral characteristics, and quality of life in women. *American Journal of Cardiology*, 1995, Vol. 75, Iss. 5, 340–343.

————. Effects of cardiac rehabilitation and exercise training programs on coronary patients with high levels of hostility. *Mayo Clinic Proceedings*, 1999, Vol. 74, Iss. 10, 959–966.

Lee, I. M., et al. Exercise and risk of stroke in male physicians. *Stroke*, 1999, Vol. 30, Iss. 1, 1–6.

Lee, I. M., R. S. Paffenbarger, Jr., and C. C. Hsieh. Time trends in physical activity among college alumni, 1962-1988. *American Journal of Epidemiology*, 1992, Vol. 135, Iss. 8, 915–925.

Lee, I. M., et al. Physical activity and coronary heart disease in women: is "no pain, no gain" passe? *Journal of the American Medical Association*, 2001, Vol. 285, Iss. 11, 1447–1454.

Lee, I. M., H. D. Sesso, and R. S. Paffenbarger, Jr. Physical activity and coronary heart disease risk in men: does the duration of exercise episodes predict risk? *Circulation*, 2000, Vol. 102, Iss. 9, 981–986.

Lewis, B. A., et al. Psychosocial mediators of physical activity behavior among adults and children. *American Journal of Preventive Medicine*, 2002, Vol. 23, Suppl. 2, 26–35.

Manson, J. E., et al. A prospective study of walking as compared with vigorous exercise in the prevention of coronary heart disease in women. *New England Journal of Medicine*, 1999, Vol. 341, Iss. 9, 650–658.

Myers, J., et al. Exercise capacity and mortality among men referred for exercise testing. *New England Journal of Medicine*, 2002, Vol. 346, Iss. 11, 793–801.

O'Connor, G. T., et al. An overview of randomized trials of rehabilitation with exercise after myocardial infarction. *Circulation*, 1989, Vol. 80, Iss. 2, 234–244.

Oldridge, N. B., et al. Cardiac rehabilitation after myocardial infarction. Combined experience of randomized clinical trials. *Journal of the American Medical Association*, 1988, Vol. 260, Iss. 7, 945–950.

Paffenbarger, R. S., Jr., S. N. Blair, and I. M. Lee. A history of physical activity, cardiovascular health and longevity: the scientific contributions of Jeremy N. Morris, DSc, DPH, FRCP. *International Journal of Epidemiology*, 2001, Vol. 30, Iss. 5, 1184–1192.

Pate, R. R., et al. Physical activity and public health. A recommendation from the Centers for Disease Control and Prevention and the American College of Sports Medicine. *Journal of the American Medical Association*, 1995, Vol. 273, Iss. 5, 402–407.

Physical activity and cardiovascular health. NIH consensus statement. National Institutes of Health, Kensington, 1995.

Physical activity and health: a report of the Surgeon General executive summary, Centers for Disease Control and Prevention, Atlanta, 1996.

Physical activity, dietary reference intakes for energy, carbohydrates, fiber, fat, protein and amino acids (macronutrients). Institute of Medicine, National Academies, Washington, D.C., 2002.

Pratt, M. Benefits of lifestyle activity vs structured exercise. *Journal of the American Medical Association*, 1999, Vol. 281, Iss. 4, 375–376.

Prevalence of recommended levels of physical activity among women—Behavioral Risk Factor Surveillance System, 1992. *Morbidity and Mortality Weekly Report*, 1995, Vol. 44, Iss. 06, 105–107, 113.

Ryan, T. J., et al. 1999 update: ACC/AHA guidelines for the management of patients with acute myocardial infarction. A report of the American College of Cardiology/American Heart Association Task Force on Practice Guidelines (Committee on Management of Acute Myocardial Infarction). *Journal of the American College of Cardiology*, 1999, Vol. 34, Iss. 3, 890–911.

Sesso, H. D., R. S. Paffenbarger, Jr., and I. M. Lee. Physical activity and coronary heart disease in men: The Harvard Alumni Health Study. *Circulation*, 2000, Vol. 102, Iss. 9, 975–980.

Shephard, R. J. Exercise in coronary heart disease. *Sports Medicine*, 1986, Vol. 3, Iss. 1, 26–49.

Shephard, R. J., and G. J. Balady. Exercise as cardiovascular therapy. *Circulation*, 1999, Vol. 99, Iss. 7, 963–972.

Sherman, S. E., et al. Comparison of past versus recent physical activity in the prevention of premature death and coronary artery disease. *American Heart Journal*, 1999, Vol. 138, Iss. 5 Pt. 1, 900–907.

Solnit, Rebecca. *Wanderlust: A History of Walking*. Viking, 2000, p. 5.

Tanasescu, M., et al. Exercise type and intensity in relation to coronary heart disease in men. *Journal of the American Medical Association*, 2002, Vol. 288, Iss. 16, 1994–2000.

Wee, C. C., et al. Physician counseling about exercise. *Journal of the American Medical Association*, 1999, Vol. 282, Iss. 16, 1583–1588.

Wei, M., et al. Relationship between low cardiorespiratory fitness and mortality in normal-weight, overweight, and obese men. *Journal of the American Medical Association*, 1999, Vol. 282, Iss. 16, 1547–1553.

Zafari, A. M., and N. K. Wenger. Secondary prevention of coronary heart disease. *Archives of Physical Medicine and Rehabilitation*, 1998, Vol. 79, Iss. 8, 1006–1017.

Strategy #4: Take Charge of Your Weight

Air, E. L., et al. Small molecule insulin mimetics reduce food intake and body weight and prevent development of obesity. *Nature Medicine*, 2002, Vol. 8, Iss. 2, 179–183.

American Heart Association. http://www.americanheart.org/presenter.jhtml?identifier=506.

Andersen, R. E., et al. Effects of lifestyle activity vs structured aerobic exercise in obese women: a randomized trial. *Journal of the American Medical Association*, 1999, Vol. 281, Iss. 4, 335–340.

Arterburn, D. E., P. K. Crane, and D. L. Veenstra. The efficacy and safety of sibutramine for weight loss. *Archives of Internal Medicine*, 2004, Vol. 164, Iss. 9, 994–1003.

Bravata, D. M., et al. Efficacy and safety of low-carbohydrate diets: a systematic review. *Journal of the American Medical Association*, 2003, Vol. 289, Iss. 14, 1837–1850.

Clinical guidelines on the identification, evaluation, and treatment of overweight and obesity in adults. National Institutes of Health. National Heart, Lung, and Blood Institute in cooperation with the National Institute of Diabetes and Digestive and Kidney Diseases, September 1998.

Clinical guidelines on the identification, evaluation, and treatment of overweight and obesity in adults—the evidence report. National Institutes of Health. *Obesity Research*, 1998, Vol. 6, Suppl. 2, 51S–209S.

De Lorenzo, A., et al. Measured and predicted resting metabolic rate in Italian males and females, aged 18–59 y. *European Journal of Clinical Nutrition*, 2001, Vol. 55, Iss. 3, 208–214.

Dunn, A. L., et al. Comparison of lifestyle and structured interventions to increase physical activity and cardiorespiratory fitness: a randomized trial. *Journal of the American Medical Association*, 1999, Vol. 281, Iss. 4, 327–334.

Foster, G. D., et al. A randomized trial of a low-carbohydrate diet for obesity. *New England Journal of Medicine*, 2003, Vol. 348, Iss. 21, 2082–2090.

Frankenfield, D. C., E. R. Muth, and W. A. Rowe. The Harris-Benedict studies of human basal metabolism: history and limitations. *Journal of the American Dietetic Association*, 1998, Vol. 98, Iss. 4, 439–445.

Garrel, D. R., N. Jobin, and L. H. de Jonge. Should we still use the Harris and Benedict equations? *Nutrition in Clinical Practice*, 1996, Vol. 11, Iss. 3, 99–103.

Glazer, G. Long-term pharmacotherapy of obesity 2000: a review of efficacy and safety. *Archives of Internal Medicine*, 2001, Vol. 161, Iss. 15, 1814–1824.

Grady, D. "Quest for Weight-Loss Drug Takes an Unusual Turn," *New York Times*, April 15, 2003, D5.

Greenway, F. L. Surgery for obesity. *Endocrinology and Metabolism Clinics of North America*, 1996, Vol. 25, Iss. 4, 1005–1027.

Gregg, E. W., et al. Intentional weight loss and death in overweight and obese U.S. adults 35 years of age and older. *Annals of Internal Medicine*, 2003, Vol. 138, Iss. 5, 383–389.

Grodstein, F., et al. Three-year follow-up of participants in a commercial weight loss program. Can you keep it off? *Archives of Internal Medicine*, 1996, Vol. 156, Iss. 12, 1302–1306.

Harris, T. B., et al. Carrying the burden of cardiovascular risk in old age: associations of weight and weight change with prevalent cardiovascular disease, risk factors, and health status in the Cardiovascular Health Study. *American Journal of Clinical Nutrition*, 1997, Vol. 66, Iss. 4, 837–844.

Heiat, A., V. Vaccarino, and H. M. Krumholz. An evidence-based assessment of federal guidelines for overweight and obesity as they apply to elderly persons. *Archives of Internal Medicine*, 2001, Vol. 161, Iss. 9, 1194–1203.

Irwin, M. L., et al. Effect of exercise on total and intra-abdominal body fat in postmenopausal women: a randomized controlled trial. *Journal of the American Medical Association*, 2003, Vol. 289, Iss. 3, 323–330.

Jakicic, J. M., et al. Effects of intermittent exercise and use of home exercise equipment on adherence, weight loss, and fitness in overweight women: a randomized trial. *Journal of the American Medical Association*, 1999, Vol. 282, Iss. 16, 1554–1560.

Krauss, R. M., et al. AHA dietary guidelines: revision 2000. A statement for healthcare professionals from the Nutrition Committee of the American Heart Association. *Circulation*, 2000, Vol. 102, Iss. 118, 2284–2299.

Mokdad, A. H., et al. Prevalence of obesity, diabetes, and obesity-related health risk factors, 2001. *Journal of the American Medical Association*, 2003, Vol. 289, Iss. 1, 76–79.

Mokdad, A. H., et al. The spread of the obesity epidemic in the United States, 1991–1998. *Journal of the American Medical Association*, 1999, Vol. 282, Iss. 16, 1519–1522.

Must, A., et al. The disease burden associated with overweight and obesity. *Journal of the American Medical Association*, 1999, Vol. 282, Iss. 16, 1523–1529.

Peeters, A., et al. Obesity in adulthood and its consequences for life expectancy: a life-table analysis. *Annals of Internal Medicine*, 2003, Vol. 138, Iss. 1, 24–32.

The practical guide: identification, evaluation, and treatment of overweight and obesity in adults. National Institutes of Health, National Heart, Lung, and Blood Institute, Bethesda, 2000.

St. Jeor, S. T., et al. Dietary protein and weight reduction: a statement for healthcare professionals from the Nutrition Committee of the Council on Nutrition, Physical Activity, and Metabolism of the American Heart Association. *Circulation*, 2001, Vol. 104, Iss. 15, 1869–1874.

Samaha, F. F., et al. A low-carbohydrate as compared with a low-fat diet in severe obesity. *New England Journal of Medicine*, 2003, Vol. 348, Iss. 21, 2074–2081.

Serdula, M. K., et al. Prevalence of attempting weight loss and strategies for controlling weight. *Journal of the American Medical Association*, 1999, Vol. 282, Iss. 14, 1353–1358.

Stern, L. et al. The effects of low-carbohydrate versus conventional weight loss diets in severely obese adults: one-year follow-up of a randomized trial. *Annals of Internal Medicine*, 2004, Vol. 140, Iss. 10, 778–785.

Stevinson, C., M. H. Pittler, and E. Ernst. Garlic for treating hyper-cholesterolemia: a meta-analysis of randomized clinical trials. *Annals of Internal Medicine*, 2000, Vol. 133, Iss. 6, 420–429.

The Surgeon General's call to action to prevent and decrease overweight and obesity. U.S. Department of Health and Human Services, 2001.

Tayback, M., S. Kumanyika, and E. Chee. Body weight as a risk factor in the elderly. *Archives of Internal Medicine*, 1990, Vol. 150, Iss. 5, 1065–1072.

Wei, M., et al. Relationship between low cardiorespiratory fitness and mortality in normal-weight, overweight, and obese men. *Journal of the American Medical Association*, 1999, Vol. 282, Iss. 16, 1547–1553.

Weinsier, R. L., et al. The etiology of obesity: relative contribution of metabolic factors, diet, and physical activity. *American Journal of Medicine*, 1998, Vol. 105, Iss. 2, 145–150.

Willett, W. C., and R. L. Leibel. Dietary fat is not a major determinant of body fat. *American Journal of Medicine*, 2002, Vol. 113, Suppl. 9B, 47S–59S.

Yanovski, S. Z., and J. A. Yanovski. Obesity. *New England Journal of Medicine*, 2002, Vol. 346, Iss. 8, 591–602.

Strategy #5: Take Charge of Your Blood Sugar

Abraira, C., et al. Cardiovascular events and correlates in the Veterans Affairs Diabetes Feasibility Trial. Veterans Affairs Cooperative Study on Glycemic Control and Complications in Type II Diabetes. *Archives of Internal Medicine*, 1997, Vol. 157, Iss. 2, 181–188.

American Diabetes Association clinical practice recommendations 2001. *Diabetes Care*, 2001, Vol. 24, Suppl 1, S1–S133.

Beckman, J. A., M. A. Creager, and P. Libby. Diabetes and atherosclerosis: epidemiology, pathophysiology, and management. *Journal of the American Medical Association*, 2002, Vol. 287, Iss. 19, 2570–2581.

Boule, N. G., et al. Effects of exercise on glycemic control and body mass in type 2 diabetes mellitus: a meta-analysis of controlled clinical trials. *Journal of the American Medical Association*, 2001, Vol. 286, Iss. 10, 1218–1227.

Buse, J. B. Overview of current therapeutic options in type 2 diabetes. Rationale for combining oral agents with insulin therapy. *Diabetes Care*, 1999, Vol. 22, Suppl. 3, C65–C70.

Colman, E., et al. Weight loss reduces abdominal fat and improves

insulin action in middle-aged and older men with impaired glucose tolerance. *Metabolism*, 1995, Vol. 44, 1502–1508.

Effect of intensive blood-glucose control with metformin on complications in overweight patients with type 2 diabetes (UKPDS
34). UK Prospective Diabetes Study (UKPDS) Group. *Lancet*,
1998, Vol. 352, Iss. 9131, 854–865.

The effect of intensive treatment of diabetes on the development
and progression of long-term complications in insulin-
dependent diabetes mellitus. The Diabetes Control and Complications Trial Research Group. *New England Journal of
Medicine*, 1993, Vol. 329, Iss. 14, 977–986.

Efficacy of atenolol and captopril in reducing risk of macrovascular
and microvascular complications in type 2 diabetes: UKPDS
39. UK Prospective Diabetes Study Group. *British Medical
Journal*, 1998, Vol. 317, Iss. 7160, 713–720.

Evidence-based nutrition principles and recommendations for the
treatment and prevention of diabetes and related complications.
American Diabetes Association. *Diabetes Care*, 2002, Vol. 25,
Iss. 1, 202–212.

Genuth, S., et al. Implications of the United Kingdom prospective
diabetes study. *Diabetes Care*, 2003, Vol. 26, Suppl. 1, S28–
S32.

Grundy, S. M., et al. Diabetes and cardiovascular disease: a statement for healthcare professionals from the American Heart Association. *Circulation*, 1999, Vol. 100, Iss. 10, 1134–1146.

Haffner, S. M. Impaired glucose tolerance, insulin resistance and
cardiovascular disease. *Diabetic Medicine*, 1997, Vol. 14, Suppl.
3, S12–S18.

————. Impaired glucose tolerance—is it relevant for cardiovascular disease? *Diabetologia*, 1997, Vol. 40, Suppl. 2, S138–S140.

Haffner, S. M., et al. Mortality from coronary heart disease in subjects with type 2 diabetes and in nondiabetic subjects with and
without prior myocardial infarction. *New England Journal of
Medicine*, 1998, Vol. 339, Iss. 4, 229–234.

Harris, M. I., et al. Prevalence of diabetes, impaired fasting glucose, and impaired glucose tolerance in U.S. adults. The Third

National Health and Nutrition Examination Survey, 1988–1994. *Diabetes Care*, 1998, Vol. 21, Iss. 4, 518–524.

Hu, F. B., et al. Diet, lifestyle, and the risk of type 2 diabetes mellitus in women. *New England Journal of Medicine*, 2001, Vol. 345, Iss. 11, 790–797.

Hu, F. B., et al. Physical activity and risk for cardiovascular events in diabetic women. *Annals of Internal Medicine*, 2001, Vol. 134, Iss. 2, 96–105.

Intensive blood-glucose control with sulphonylureas or insulin compared with conventional treatment and risk of complications in patients with type 2 diabetes (UKPDS 33). UK Prospective Diabetes Study (UKPDS) Group. *Lancet*, 1998, Vol. 352, Iss. 9131, 837–853.

Knowler, W. C., et al. Reduction in the incidence of type 2 diabetes with lifestyle intervention or metformin. *New England Journal of Medicine*, 2002, Vol. 346, Iss. 6, 393–403.

Larger, E., et al. Insulin therapy does not itself induce weight gain in patients with type 2 diabetes. *Diabetes Care*, 2001, Vol. 24, Iss. 10, 1849–1850.

Ludwig, D. S. The glycemic index: physiological mechanisms relating to obesity, diabetes, and cardiovascular disease. *Journal of the American Medical Association*, 2002, Vol. 287, Iss. 18, 2414–2423.

Mokdad, A. H., et al. Diabetes trends in the U.S.: 1990–1998. *Diabetes Care*, 2000, Vol. 23, Iss. 9, 1278–1283.

O'Brien, T., T. T. Nguyen, and B. R. Zimmerman. Hyperlipidemia and diabetes mellitus. *Mayo Clinic Proceedings*, 1998, Vol. 73, Iss. 10, 969–976.

Reaven, G. M., H. Lithell, and L. Landsberg. Hypertension and associated metabolic abnormalities—the role of insulin resistance and the sympathoadrenal system. *New England Journal of Medicine*, 1996, Vol. 334, Iss. 6, 374–381.

Robertson, R. P., et al. Pancreas transplantation for patients with type 1 diabetes. *Diabetes Care*, 2003, Vol. 26, Suppl. 1, S120.

Rosenfeld, L. Insulin: discovery and controversy. *Clinical Chemistry*, 2002, Vol. 48, Iss. 12, 2270–2288.

Screening for type 2 diabetes. American Diabetes Association. *Diabetes Care*, 2003, Vol. 26, Suppl. 1, S21–S24.

Standards of medical care for patients with diabetes mellitus. American Diabetes Association. *Diabetes Care*, 2003, Vol. 26, Suppl. 1, S33–S50.

Tight blood pressure control and risk of macrovascular and microvascular complications in type 2 diabetes: UKPDS 38. UK Prospective Diabetes Study Group. *British Medical Journal*, 1998, Vol. 317, Iss. 7160, 703–713.

Wilson, P.W. Diabetes mellitus and coronary heart disease. *American Journal of Kidney Disease*, 1998, Vol. 32, 5 Suppl. 3, S89–S100.

Yki-Jarvinen, H. Combination therapies with insulin in type 2 diabetes. *Diabetes Care*, 2001, Vol. 24, Iss. 4, 758–767.

Strategy #6: Take Charge of Your Smoking

Abbot, N.C., et al. Hypnotherapy for smoking cessation. *Cochrane Database System Review*, 2000, Vol. 2, CD001008.

Cigarette smoking among adults—United States, 1999. *Morbidity and Mortality Weekly Report*, 2001, Vol. 50, Iss. 40, 869–873.

A clinical practice guideline for treating tobacco use and dependence: A U.S. Public Health Service report. The Tobacco Use and Dependence Clinical Practice Guideline Panel, Staff, and Consortium Representatives. *Journal of the American Medical Association*, 2000, Vol. 283, Iss. 24, 3244–3254.

David, S., T. Lancaster, and L.F. Stead. Opioid antagonists for smoking cessation. *Cochrane Database System Review*, 2001, Vol. 3, CD003086.

Fiore, M.C., et al. Clinical practice guideline: treating tobacco use and dependence. U.S. Department of Health and Human Services, June 2000.

Gourlay, S.G., L.F. Stead, and N.L. Benowitz. Clonidine for smoking cessation. *Cochrane Database System Review*, 2000, Vol. 2, CD000058.

Hajek, P., and L.F. Stead. Aversive smoking for smoking cessation. *Cochrane Database System Review*, 2000, Vol. 2, CD000546.

Hays, J.T., et al. Sustained-release bupropion for pharmacologic relapse prevention after smoking cessation. A randomized, controlled trial. *Annals of Internal Medicine*, 2001, Vol. 135, Iss. 6, 423–433.

Howard, G., et al. Cigarette smoking and progression of atherosclerosis: The Atherosclerosis Risk in Communities (ARIC) study. *Journal of the American Medical Association*, 1998, Vol. 279, Iss. 2, 119–124.

Hughes, J.R., L.F. Stead, and T. Lancaster. Antidepressants for smoking cessation. *Cochrane Database System Review*, 2000, Vol. 4, CD000031.

———. Anxiolytics and antidepressants for smoking cessation. *Cochrane Database System Review*, 2000, Vol. 2, CD000031.

Jorenby, D.E. Smoking cessation strategies for the 21st century. *Circulation*, 2001, Vol. 104, Iss. 11, E51–E52.

Joseph, A.M., et al. The safety of transdermal nicotine as an aid to smoking cessation in patients with cardiac disease. *New England Journal of Medicine*, 1996, Vol. 335, Iss. 24, 1792–1798.

Krumholz, H.M., et al. Cost-effectiveness of a smoking cessation program after myocardial infarction. *Journal of the American College of Cardiology*, 1993, Vol. 22, Iss. 6, 1697–1702.

Lancaster, T., and L.F. Stead. Individual behavioural counselling for smoking cessation. *Cochrane Database System Review*, 2000, Vol. 2, CD001292.

———. Mecamylamine (a nicotine antagonist) for smoking cessation. Cochrane Database System Review, 2000, Vol. 2, CD001009.

———. Self-help interventions for smoking cessation. *Cochrane Database System Review*, 2000, Vol. 2, CD001118.

———. Silver acetate for smoking cessation. *Cochrane Database System Review*, 2000, Vol. 2, CD000191.

Perspectives in disease prevention and health promotion-smoking attributable mortality and years of potential life lost—United States, 1984. Centers for Disease Control and Prevention. *Morbidity and Mortality Weekly Report*, 1997, Vol. 46, Iss. 20, 444–451.

Rea, T. D., et al. Smoking status and risk for recurrent coronary events after myocardial infarction. *Annals of Internal Medicine*, 2002, Vol. 137, Iss. 6, 494–500.

Rice, V. H. Nursing intervention and smoking cessation: a meta-analysis. *Heart and Lung*, 1999, Vol. 28, Iss. 6, 438–454.

Rice, V. H., and L. F. Stead. Nursing interventions for smoking cessation. *Cochrane Database System Review*, 2001, Vol. 3, CD001188.

Rigotti, N. A. Clinical practice. Treatment of tobacco use and dependence. *New England Journal of Medicine*, 2002, Vol. 346, Iss. 7, 506–512.

Schroeder, S. A. Conflicting dispatches from the tobacco wars. *New England Journal of Medicine*, 2002, Vol. 347, Iss. 14, 1106–1109.

Silagy, C., and L. F. Stead. Physician advice for smoking cessation. *Cochrane Database System Review*, 2001, Vol. 2, CD000165.

Smith, S. C., Jr., et al. AHA/ACC Scientific Statement: AHA/ACC guidelines for preventing heart attack and death in patients with atherosclerotic cardiovascular disease: 2001 update: a statement for healthcare professionals from the American Heart Association and the American College of Cardiology. *Circulation*, 2001, Vol. 104, Iss. 13, 1577–1579.

Stead, L. F, and T. Lancaster. Group behaviour therapy programmes for smoking cessation. *Cochrane Database System Review*, 2000, Vol. 2, CD001007.

———. Telephone counselling for smoking cessation. *Cochrane Database System Review*, 2001, Vol. 2, CD002850.

Stead, L. F., and J. R. Hughes. Lobeline for smoking cessation. *Cochrane Database System Review*, 2000, Vol. 2, CD000124.

Surgeon General's five-day plan to get ready, www.surgeongeneral.gov/tobacco.

Ussher, M. H., et al. Does exercise aid smoking cessation? A systematic review. *Addiction*, 2000, Vol. 95, Iss. 2, 199–208.

Ussher, M. H., et al. Exercise interventions for smoking cessation. *Cochrane Database System Review*, 2000, Vol. 3, CD002295.

Werner, R. M., and T. A. Pearson. What's so passive about passive smoking? Secondhand smoke as a cause of atherosclerotic disease. *Journal of the American Medical Association*, 1998, Vol. 279, Iss. 2, 157–158.

White, A. R., H. Rampes, and E. Ernst. Acupuncture for smoking cessation. *Cochrane Database System Review*, 2000, Vol. 2, CD000009.

White, A. R., K. L. Resch, and E. Ernst. A meta-analysis of acupuncture techniques for smoking cessation. *Tobacco Control*, 1999, Vol. 8, Iss. 4, 393–397.

Zhu, S. H., et al. Evidence of real-world effectiveness of a telephone quitline for smokers. *New England Journal of Medicine*, 2002, Vol. 347, Iss. 14, 1087–1093.

Strategy #7: Take Charge of Your Medications

Baron, J. A., et al. A randomized trial of aspirin to prevent colorectal adenomas. *New England Journal of Medicine*, 2003, Vol. 348, Iss. 10, 891–899.

Braunwald, E., et al. ACC/AHA 2002 guideline update for the management of patients with unstable angina and non-ST-segment elevation myocardial infarction—summary article: a report of the American College of Cardiology/American Heart Association Task Force on Practice Guidelines (Committee on the Management of Patients with Unstable Angina). *Journal of the American College of Cardiology*, 2002, Vol. 40, Iss. 7, 1366–1374.

Collaborative meta-analysis of randomised trials of antiplatelet therapy for prevention of death, myocardial infarction, and stroke in high risk patients. *British Medical Journal*, 2002, Vol. 324, Iss. 6921, 71–86.

Collaborative overview of randomised trials of antiplatelet therapy—I: Prevention of death, myocardial infarction, and stroke by prolonged antiplatelet therapy in various categories of patients. Antiplatelet Trialists' Collaboration. *British Medical Journal*, 1994, Vol. 308, Iss. 6921, 81–106.

Collaborative overview of randomised trials of antiplatelet therapy—II: Maintenance of vascular graft or arterial patency by antiplatelet therapy. Antiplatelet Trialists' Collaboration. *British Medical Journal*, 1994, Vol. 308, Iss. 6922, 159–168.

Final report on the aspirin component of the ongoing Physicians' Health Study. Steering Committee of the Physicians' Health Study Research Group. *New England Journal of Medicine*, 1989, Vol. 321, Iss. 3, 129–135.

Freedman, J. E., et al. Select flavonoids and whole juice from purple grapes inhibit platelet function and enhance nitric oxide release. *Circulation*, 2001, Vol. 103, Iss. 23, 2792–2798.

Gamble, E. Cardioselective beta blockers do not cause adverse respiratory effects in mild to moderate reactive airway disease. *Thorax*, 2003, Vol. 58, 142.

Gum, P. A., et al. Profile and prevalence of aspirin resistance in patients with cardiovascular disease. *American Journal of Cardiology*, 2001, Vol. 88, Iss. 3, 230–235.

Hennekens, C. H., M. L. Dyken, and V. Fuster. Aspirin as a therapeutic agent in cardiovascular disease: a statement for healthcare professionals from the American Heart Association. *Circulation*, 1997, Vol. 96, Iss. 8, 2751–2753.

Hurlen, M., et al. Warfarin, aspirin, or both after myocardial infarction. *New England Journal of Medicine*, 2002, Vol. 347, Iss. 13, 969–974.

Kelly, J. P., et al. Risk of aspirin-associated major upper-gastrointestinal bleeding with enteric-coated or buffered product. *Lancet*, 1996, Vol. 348, Iss. 9039, 1413–1416.

Ko, D. T., et al. Beta-blocker therapy and symptoms of depression, fatigue, and sexual dysfunction. *Journal of the American Medical Association*, 2002, Vol. 288, Iss. 3, 351–357.

Ko, D., et al. Nonsteroidal antiinflammatory drugs after acute myocardial infarction. *American Heart Journal*, 2002, Vol. 143, Iss. 3, 475–481.

MacDonald, T. M., and L. Wei. Effect of ibuprofen on cardioprotective effect of aspirin. *Lancet*, 2003, Vol. 361, Iss. 9357, 573–574.

Maggioni, A. P. Secondary prevention: improving outcomes following myocardial infarction. *Heart*, 2000, Vol. 84, Suppl. 1, i5–i7, discussion i50.

Mangano, D. T. Aspirin and mortality from coronary bypass surgery. *New England Journal of Medicine*, 2002, Vol. 347, Iss. 17, 1309–1317.

Mann, Charles. *The Aspirin Wars: Money, Medicine, and 100 Years of Rampant Competition*. Alfred A. Knopf, 1991.

Mueller, R. L., and S. Scheidt. History of drugs for thrombotic disease. Discovery, development, and directions for the future. *Circulation*, 1994, Vol 89, Iss. 1, 432–449.

O'Keefe, J. H., et al. Should an angiotensin-converting enzyme inhibitor be standard therapy for patients with atherosclerotic disease? *Journal of the American College of Cardiology*, 2001, Vol. 37, Iss. 1, 1–8.

Pepine, C. J. Aspirin and newer orally active antiplatelet agents in the treatment of the post-myocardial infarction patient. *Journal of the American College of Cardiology*, 1998, Vol. 32, Iss. 4, 1126–1128.

Pfeffer, M. A. ACE inhibition in acute myocardial infarction. *New England Journal of Medicine*, 1995, Vol. 332, Iss. 2, 118–120.

Pfeffer, M. A., et al. Effect of captopril on mortality and morbidity in patients with left ventricular dysfunction after myocardial infarction. Results of the survival and ventricular enlargement trial. The SAVE Investigators. *New England Journal of Medicine*, 1992, Vol. 327, Iss. 10, 669–677.

Pfeffer, M. A., et al. The continuation of the Prevention of Events with Angiotensin-Converting Enzyme Inhibition (PEACE) trial. *American Heart Journal*, 2001, Vol. 142, Iss. 3, 375–377.

A randomised, blinded, trial of clopidogrel versus aspirin in patients at risk of ischaemic events (CAPRIE). CAPRIE Steering Committee. *Lancet*, 1996, Vol. 348, Iss. 9038, 1329–1339.

Randomised trial of intravenous streptokinase, oral aspirin, both, or neither among 17,187 cases of suspected acute myocardial infarction: ISIS-2. ISIS-2 (Second International Study of Infarct

Survival) Collaborative Group. *Lancet*, 1988, Vol. 2, Iss. 8607, 349–360.

Ray, W. A., et al. Non-steroidal anti-inflammatory drugs and risk of serious coronary heart disease: an observational cohort study. *Lancet*, 2002, Vol. 359, Iss. 9301, 118–123.

Sabesin, S. M., et al. Comparative evaluation of gastrointestinal intolerance produced by plain and tri-buffered aspirin tablets. *American Journal of Gastroenterology*, 1988, Vol. 83, Iss. 11, 1220–1225.

Salpeter, S. R., T. M. Ormiston, and E. E. Salpeter. Cardioselective beta-blockers in patients with reactive airway disease: a meta-analysis. *Annals of Internal Medicine*, 2002, Vol. 137, Iss. 9, 715–725.

Sandler, R. S., et al. A randomized trial of aspirin to prevent colorectal adenomas in patients with previous colorectal cancer. *New England Journal of Medicine*, 2003, Vol. 348, Iss. 10, 883–890.

Savon, J. J., et al. Gastrointestinal blood loss with low dose (325 mg) plain and enteric-coated aspirin administration. *American Journal of Gastroenterology*, 1995, Vol. 90, Iss. 4, 581–585.

Sharis, P. J., C. P. Cannon, and J. Loscalzo. The antiplatelet effects of ticlopidine and clopidogrel. *Annals of Internal Medicine*, 1998, Vol. 129, Iss. 5, 394–405.

Smith, P., H. Arnesen, and M. Abdelnoor. Effects of long-term anticoagulant therapy in subgroups after acute myocardial infarction. *Archives of Internal Medicine*, 1992, Vol. 152, Iss. 5, 993–997.

Sorensen, H. T., et al. Risk of upper gastrointestinal bleeding associated with use of low-dose aspirin. *American Journal of Gastroenterology*, 2000, Vol. 95, Iss. 9, 2218–2224.

Steinhubl, S. R., et al. Early and sustained dual oral antiplatelet therapy following percutaneous coronary intervention: a randomized controlled trial. *Journal of the American Medical Association*, 2002, Vol. 288, Iss. 19, 2411–2420.

Timolol-induced reduction in mortality and reinfarction in patients surviving acute myocardial infarction. *New England Journal of Medicine*, 1981, Vol. 304, Iss. 14, 801–807.

Valli, G., and E. G. Giardina. Benefits, adverse effects and drug interactions of herbal therapies with cardiovascular effects. *Journal of the American College of Cardiology,* 2002, Vol. 39, Iss. 7, 1083–1095.

van Es, R. F., et al. Aspirin and coumadin after acute coronary syndromes (the ASPECT-2 study): a randomised controlled trial. *Lancet,* 2002, Vol. 360, Iss. 9327, 109–113.

Vane, J. R. The history of inhibitors of angiotensin converting enzyme. *Journal of Physiology and Pharmacology,* 1999, Vol. 50, Iss. 4, 489–498.

Viscoli, C. M., R. I. Horwitz, and B. H. Singer. Beta-blockers after myocardial infarction: influence of first-year clinical course on long-term effectiveness. *Annals of Internal Medicine,* 1993, Vol. 118, Iss. 2, 99–105.

Yusuf, S., et al. Beta blockade during and after myocardial infarction: an overview of the randomized trials. *Progress in Cardiovascular Diseases,* 1985, Vol. 27, Iss. 5, 335–371.

Yusuf, S., et al. Effects of an angiotensin-converting-enzyme inhibitor, ramipril, on cardiovascular events in high-risk patients. The Heart Outcomes Prevention Evaluation Study Investigators. *New England Journal of Medicine,* 2000, Vol. 342, Iss. 3, 145–153.

Yusuf, S., et al Effects of clopidogrel in addition to aspirin in patients with acute coronary syndromes without ST-segment elevation. *New England Journal of Medicine,* 2001, Vol. 345, Iss. 7, 494–502.

Zandi, P. P., et al. Reduced incidence of AD with NSAID but not H2 receptor antagonists: the Cache County Study. *Neurology,* 2002, Vol. 59, Iss. 6, 880–886.

Chapter 3. Beyond the Key Strategies

Managing Your Diet

Albert, C. M., et al. Blood levels of long-chain n-3 fatty acids and the risk of sudden death. *New England Journal of Medicine,* 2002, Vol. 346, Iss. 15, 1113–1118.

Albert, C. M., et al. Nut consumption and decreased risk of sudden cardiac death in the Physicians' Health Study. *Archives of Internal Medicine*, 2002, Vol. 162, Iss. 12, 1382–1387.

Anderson, J. W., et al. Meta-analysis of the effects of soy protein intake on serum lipids. *New England Journal of Medicine*, 1995, Vol. 333, Iss. 5, 276–282.

Ascherio, A., et al. Dietary fat and risk of coronary heart disease in men: cohort follow up study in the United States. *British Medical Journal*, 1996, Vol. 313, Iss. 7049, 84–90.

Burr, M. L., et al. Effects of changes in fat, fish, and fibre intakes on death and myocardial reinfarction: diet and reinfarction trial (DART). *Lancet*, 1989, Vol. 2, Iss. 8666, 757–761.

Byers, T., et al. American Cancer Society guidelines on nutrition and physical activity for cancer prevention: reducing the risk of cancer with healthy food choices and physical activity. *CA: A Cancer Journal for Clinicians*, 2002, Vol. 52, Iss. 2, 92–119.

de Lorgeril, M., et al. Mediterranean diet, traditional risk factors, and the rate of cardiovascular complications after myocardial infarction: final report of the Lyon Diet Heart Study. *Circulation*, 1999, Vol. 99, Iss. 6, 779–785.

Dietary fat consensus statements. *American Journal of Medicine*, 2002, Vol. 113, Suppl. 9B, 5S–8S.

Dietary reference intakes for energy, carbohydrate, fiber, fat, fatty acids, cholesterol, protein, and amino acids. Washington, D.C.: Institute of Medicine of the National Academies; 2002.

Dietary supplementation with n-3 polyunsaturated fatty acids and vitamin E after myocardial infarction: results of the GISSI-Prevenzione trial. Gruppo Italiano per lo Studio della Sopravvivenza nell'Infarto Miocardico. *Lancet*, 1999, Vol. 354, Iss. 9177, 447–455.

Duffy, S. J., et al. Short- and long-term black tea consumption reverses endothelial dysfunction in patients with coronary artery disease. *Circulation*, 2001, Vol. 104, Iss. 2, 151–156.

Duffy, S. J., et al. Effect of acute and chronic tea consumption on platelet aggregation in patients with coronary artery disease. *Ar-*

teriosclerosis, Thrombosis and Vascular Biology, 2001, Vol. 21, Iss. 6, 1084–1089.

Evaluation of certain food additives and contaminants. Forty-sixth report of the Joint FAO/WHO Expert Committee on Food Additives. World Health Organization Technical Reporting Service, 1997, Vol. 868, 1–69.

Facts about the DASH diet. National Institutes of Health, National Heart, Lung, and Blood Institute, Bethesda, 1998.

Foreyt, J. P., and W. S. Poston. Consensus view on the role of dietary fat and obesity. *American Journal of Medicine,* 2002, Vol. 113, Suppl. 9B, 60S–62S.

Geleijnse, J. M., et al. Tea flavonoids may protect against atherosclerosis: the Rotterdam Study. *Archives of Internal Medicine,* 1999, Vol. 159, Iss. 18, 2170–2174.

He, K., et al. Fish consumption and risk of stroke in men. *Journal of the American Medical Association,* 2002, Vol. 288, Iss. 24, 3130–3136.

Hites, R. A., et al. Global assessment of organic contaminants in farmed salmon. *Science,* 2004, Vol. 303, Iss. 5655, 226–229.

Holub, B. J. Clinical nutrition: 4. Omega-3 fatty acids in cardiovascular care. *Canadian Medical Association Journal,* 2002, Vol. 166, Iss. 5, 608–615.

Hu, F. B., and W. C. Willett. Optimal diets for prevention of coronary heart disease. *Journal of the American Medical Association,* 2002, Vol. 288, Iss. 20, 2569–2578.

Hu, F. B., et al. Fish and omega-3 fatty acid intake and risk of coronary heart disease in women. *Journal of the American Medical Association,* 2002, Vol. 287, Iss. 14, 1815–1821.

Hu, F. B., et al. Frequent nut consumption and risk of coronary heart disease in women: prospective cohort study. *British Medical Journal,* 1998, Vol. 317, Iss. 7169, 1341–1345.

Jenkins, D. J., et al. Dose response of almonds on coronary heart disease risk factors: blood lipids, oxidized low-density lipoproteins, lipoprotein(a), homocysteine, and pulmonary nitric oxide. *Circulation,* 2002, Vol. 106, Iss. 11, 1327–1332.

Jiang, R., et al. Nut and peanut butter consumption and risk of type 2 diabetes in women. *Journal of the American Medical Association*, 2002, Vol. 288, Iss. 20, 2554–2560.

Joshipura K. J., et al. The effect of fruit and vegetable intake on risk for coronary heart disease. *Annals of Internal Medicine*, 2001, Vol. 134, Iss. 12, 1106–1114.

Krauss, R. M., et al. AHA Dietary Guidelines: revision 2000: a statement for healthcare professionals from the Nutrition Committee of the American Heart Association. *Circulation*, 2000, Vol. 102, Iss. 18, 2284–2299.

Kris-Etherton, P. M., W. S. Harris, and L. J. Appel. Fish consumption, fish oil, omega-3 fatty acids, and cardiovascular disease. *Circulation*, 2002, Vol. 106, Iss. 21, 2747–2757.

Liu, S., et al. Whole-grain consumption and risk of coronary heart disease: results from the Nurses' Health Study. *American Journal of Clinical Nutrition*, 1999, Vol. 70, Iss. 3, 412–419.

Marchioli, R., et al. Early protection against sudden death by n-3 polyunsaturated fatty acids after myocardial infarction: time-course analysis of the results of the Gruppo Italiano per lo Studio della Sopravvivenza nell'Infarto Miocardico (GISSI)-Prevenzione. *Circulation*, 2002, Vol. 105, Iss. 16, 1897–1903.

Nielsen, S. J., and B. M. Popkin. Patterns and trends in food portion sizes, 1977–1998. *Journal of the American Medical Association*, 2003, Vol. 289, Iss. 4, 450–453.

Ornish, D., et al. Intensive lifestyle changes for reversal of coronary heart disease. *Journal of the American Medical Association*, 1998, Vol. 280, Iss. 23, 2001–2007.

Pereira, M. A., et al. Dietary fiber and risk of coronary heart disease. *Archives of Internal Medicine*, 2004, Vol. 164, Iss. 4, 370–376.

Sesso, H. D., et al. Coffee and tea intake and the risk of myocardial infarction. *American Journal of Epidemiology*, 1999, Vol. 149, Iss. 2, 162–167.

Stevinson, C., M. H. Pittler, and E. Ernst. Garlic for treating hypercholesterolemia. A meta-analysis of randomized clinical trials. *Annals of Internal Medicine*, 2000, Vol. 133, Iss. 6, 420–429.

Titan, S. M., et al. Frequency of eating and concentrations of serum cholesterol in the Norfolk population of the European Prospective Investigation into Cancer (EPIC-Norfolk): cross sectional study. *British Medical Journal*, 2001, Vol. 323, Iss. 7324, 1286–1288.

Willett, W. C., and M. J. Stampfer. Rebuilding the food pyramid. *Scientific American*, 2003, Vol. 288, Iss. 1, 64–71.

Wylie-Rosett, J. Fat substitutes and health: an advisory from the Nutrition Committee of the American Heart Association. *Circulation*, 2002, Vol. 105, Iss. 23, 2800–2804.

Consuming Alcohol

Albert, M. A., R. J. Glynn, and P. M. Ridker. Alcohol consumption and plasma concentration of C-reactive protein. *Circulation*, 2003, Vol. 107, Iss. 3, 443–447.

Berger, K., et al. Light-to-moderate alcohol consumption and risk of stroke among U.S. male physicians. *New England Journal of Medicine*, 1999, Vol. 341, Iss. 21, 1557–1564.

Corder, R., et al. Endothelin-1 synthesis reduced by red wine. *Nature*, 2001, Vol. 414, Iss. 6866, 863–864.

Gronbaek, M., et al. Type of alcohol consumed and mortality from all causes, coronary heart disease, and cancer. *Annals of Internal Medicine*, 2000, Vol. 133, Iss. 6, 411–419.

Miyagi, Y., K. Miwa, and H. Inoue. Inhibition of human low-density lipoprotein oxidation by flavonoids in red wine and grape juice. *American Journal of Cardiology*, 1997, Vol. 80, Iss. 12, 1627–1631.

Mukamal, K. J., et al. Roles of drinking pattern and type of alcohol consumed in coronary heart disease in men. *New England Journal of Medicine*, 2003, Vol. 348, Iss. 2, 109–118.

Naimi, T. S., et al. Binge drinking among US adults. *Journal of the American Medical Association*, 2003, Vol. 289, Iss. 1, 70–75.

Reynolds, K., et al. Alcohol consumption and risk of stroke: a meta-analysis. *Journal of the American Medical Association*, 2003, Vol. 289, Iss. 5, 579–588.

Rimm, E. B., et al. Moderate alcohol intake and lower risk of coronary heart disease: meta-analysis of effects on lipids and haemostatic factors. *British Medical Journal*, 1999, Vol. 319, Iss. 7224, 1523–1528.

Stampfer, M., and E. Rimm. Why heart disease mortality is low in France. Commentary: alcohol and other dietary factors may be important. *British Medical Journal*, 1999, Vol. 318, Iss. 7196, 1476–1477.

Walsh, C. R., et al. Alcohol consumption and risk for congestive heart failure in the Framingham Heart Study. *Annals of Internal Medicine*, 2002, Vol. 136, Iss. 3, 181–191.

Wannamethee, S. G., and A. G. Shaper. Taking up regular drinking in middle age: effect on major coronary heart disease events and mortality. *Heart*, 2002, Vol. 87, Iss. 1, 32–36.

Taking Vitamins and Other Supplements

Ascherio, A., et al. Relation of consumption of vitamin E, vitamin C, and carotenoids to risk for stroke among men in the United States. *Annals of Internal Medicine*, 1999, Vol. 130, Iss. 12, 963–970.

Bostom, A. G., et al. Power Shortage: clinical trials testing the "homocysteine hypothesis" against a background of folic acid-fortified cereal grain flour. *Annals of Internal Medicine*, 2001, Vol. 135, Iss. 2, 133–137.

Brown, B. G., et al. Simvastatin and niacin, antioxidant vitamins, or the combination for the prevention of coronary disease. *New England Journal of Medicine*, 2001, Vol. 345, Iss. 22, 1583–1592.

Corrigan, J. J., Jr., and L. L. Ulfers. Effect of vitamin E on prothrombin levels in warfarin-induced vitamin K deficiency. *American Journal of Clinical Nutrition*, 1981, Vol. 34, Iss. 9, 1701–1705.

Dietary supplements; vitamin sales rose 50% since 1994, report says. *Chicago Tribune* 1999, January 29, 7.

Jacques, P. F., et al. The effect of folic acid fortification on plasma folate and total homocysteine concentrations. *New England Journal of Medicine*, 1999, Vol. 340, Iss. 19, 1449–1454.

Kim, J. M., and R. H. White. Effect of vitamin E on the anticoagulant response to warfarin. *American Journal of Cardiology*, 1996, Vol. 77, Iss. 7, 545–546.

Kolata, G. Vitamins: more may be too many. *New York Times* 2003, April 29, 1.

Mayer, C. E. Rite Aid, GNC form an alliance; nutrition outlets coming to drugstores. *Washington Post*, 1999, January 8, F03.

MRC/BHF Heart Protection Study of antioxidant vitamin supplementation in 20,536 high-risk individuals: a randomised placebo-controlled trial. *Lancet*, 2002, Vol. 360, Iss. 9326, 23–33.

Nutrition Examination Survey (1991–1994): population reference ranges and contribution of vitamin status to high serum concentrations. *Annals of Internal Medicine*, 1999, Vol. 131, Iss. 5, 331–339.

Pruthi, S., T. G. Allison, and D. D. Hensrud. Vitamin E supplementation in the prevention of coronary heart disease. *Mayo Clinic Proceedings*, 2001, Vol. 76, Iss. 11, 1131–1136.

Schnyder, G., et al. Effect of homocysteine-lowering therapy with folic acid, vitamin B(12), and vitamin B(6) on clinical outcome after percutaneous coronary intervention: the Swiss Heart study: a randomized controlled trial. *Journal of the American Medical Association*, 2002, Vol. 288, Iss. 8, 973–979.

Selhub, J., et al. Serum total homocysteine concentrations in the third National Health and Nutrition Examination Survey (1991–1994): population reference ranges and contribution of vitamin status to high serum concentrations. *Annals of Internal Medicine*, 1999, Vol. 131, Iss. 5, 331–339.

Willett, W. C., and M. J. Stampfer. Clinical practice. What vitamins should I be taking, doctor? *New England Journal of Medicine*, 2001, Vol. 345, Iss. 25, 1819–1824.

Yusuf, S., et al. Vitamin E supplementation and cardiovascular events in high-risk patients. The Heart Outcomes Prevention Evaluation Study Investigators. *New England Journal of Medicine*, 2000, Vol. 342, Iss. 3, 154–160.

Reducing Stress

Benson, H., J. F. Beary, and M. P. Carol. The relaxation response. *Psychiatry*, 1974, Vol. 37, Iss. 1, 37–46.

Benson, H., J. B. Kotch, and K. D. Crassweller. Stress and hypertension: interrelations and management. *Cardiovascular Clinics*, 1978, Vol. 9, Iss. 1, 113–124.

Bernardi, L., et al. Effect of rosary prayer and yoga mantras on autonomic cardiovascular rhythms: comparative study. *British Medical Journal*, 2001, Vol. 323, Iss. 1, 1446–1449.

Blumenthal, J. A., et al. Usefulness of psychosocial treatment of mental stress-induced myocardial ischemia in men. *American Journal of Cardiology*, 2002, Vol. 89, Iss. 2, 164–168.

Coronary-prone behavior and coronary heart disease: a critical review. The Review Panel on Coronary-prone Behavior and Coronary Heart Disease. *Circulation*, 1981, Vol. 63, Iss. 6, 1199–1215.

Esch, T., et al. Stress in cardiovascular diseases. *Medical Science Monitor*, 2002, Vol. 8, Iss. 5, RA93–RA101.

Hemingway, H., and M. Marmot. Evidence based cardiology: psychosocial factors in the aetiology and prognosis of coronary heart disease. Systematic review of prospective cohort studies. *British Medical Journal*, 1999, Vol. 318, Iss. 7196, 1460–1467.

Johnston, D. W., D. G. Cook, and A. G. Shaper. Type A behaviour and ischaemic heart disease in middle aged British men. *British Medical Journal (Clinical Research Edition)*, 1987, Vol. 295, Iss. 6590, 86–89.

Kaplan, G. A., and J. E. Keil. Socioeconomic factors and cardiovascular disease: a review of the literature. *Circulation*, 1993, Vol. 88, Iss. 4 Pt. 1, 1973–1998.

Kario, K., et al. Factors associated with the occurrence and magnitude of earthquake-induced increases in blood pressure. *American Journal of Medicine*, 2001, Vol. 111, Iss. 5, 379–384.

Kubzansky, L. D., et al. Anxiety and coronary heart disease: a synthesis of epidemiological, psychological, and experimental evidence. *Annals of Behavioral Medicine*, 1998, Vol. 20, Iss. 2, 47–58.

Leor, J., W. K. Poole, and R. A. Kloner. Sudden cardiac death triggered by an earthquake. *New England Journal of Medicine*, 1996, Vol. 334, Iss. 7, 413–419.

Parati, G., et al. Cardiovascular effects of an earthquake: direct evidence by ambulatory blood pressure monitoring. *Hypertension*, 2001, Vol. 38, Iss. 5, 1093–1095.

van Montfrans, G. A., et al. Relaxation therapy and continuous ambulatory blood pressure in mild hypertension: a controlled study. *British Medical Journal*, 1990, Vol. 300, Iss. 6736, 1368–1372.

Using Hormone Therapy

Anderson, G. L., et al. Effects of conjugated equine estrogen in postmenopausal women with hysterectomy: the Women's Health Initiative randomized controlled trial. *Journal of the American Medical Association*, 2004, Vol. 291, Iss. 14, 1701–1712.

Grady, D., et al. Cardiovascular disease outcomes during 6.8 years of hormone therapy: Heart and Estrogen/progestin Replacement Study follow-up (HERS II). *Journal of the American Medical Association*, 2002, Vol. 288, Iss. 1, 49–57.

Grady, D. Postmenopausal hormones—therapy for symptoms only. *New England Journal of Medicine*, 2003, Vol. 348, Iss. 19, 1835–1837.

Grodstein, F., J. E. Manson, and M. J. Stampfer. Postmenopausal hormone use and secondary prevention of coronary events in the Nurses' Health Study. A prospective, observational study. *Annals of Internal Medicine*, 2001, Vol. 135, Iss. 1, 1–8.

Hays, J., et al. Effects of estrogen plus progestin on health-related quality of life. *New England Journal of Medicine*, 2003, Vol. 348, Iss. 19, 1839–1854.

Hodis, H. N., et al. Estrogen in the prevention of atherosclerosis. A randomized, double-blind, placebo-controlled trial. *Annals of Internal Medicine*, 2001, Vol. 135, Iss. 11, 939–953.

Hulley, S., et al. Noncardiovascular disease outcomes during 6.8 years of hormone therapy: Heart and Estrogen/progestin Replacement Study follow-up (HERS II). *Journal of the American Medical Association*, 2002, Vol. 288, Iss. 1, 58–66.

Hulley, S., et al. Randomized trial of estrogen plus progestin for secondary prevention of coronary heart disease in post-menopausal women. Heart and Estrogen/progestin Replacement Study (HERS) Research Group. *Journal of the American Medical Association*, 1998, Vol. 280, Iss. 7, 605–613.

Humphrey, L. L., B. K. Chan, and H. C. Sox. Postmenopausal hormone replacement therapy and the primary prevention of cardiovascular disease. *Annals of Internal Medicine*, 2002, Vol. 137, Iss. 4, 273–284.

Koh, K. K., et al. Statin attenuates increase in C-reactive protein during estrogen replacement therapy in postmenopausal women. *Circulation*, 2002, Vol. 105, Iss. 13, 1531–1533.

Manson, J. E., and K. A. Martin. Clinical practice. Postmenopausal hormone-replacement therapy. *New England Journal of Medicine*, 2001, Vol. 345, Iss. 1, 34–40.

Miller, J., B. K. Chan, and H. D. Nelson. Postmenopausal estrogen replacement and risk for venous thromboembolism: a systematic review and meta-analysis for the U.S. Preventive Services Task Force. *Annals of Internal Medicine*, 2002, Vol. 136, Iss. 9, 680–690.

Mosca, L., et al. Hormone replacement therapy and cardiovascular disease: a statement for healthcare professionals from the American Heart Association. *Circulation*, 2001, Vol. 104, Iss. 4, 499–503.

Nelson, H. D. Assessing benefits and harms of hormone replacement therapy: clinical applications. *Journal of the American Medical Association*, 2002, Vol. 288, Iss. 7, 882–884.

Nelson, H. D., et al. Postmenopausal hormone replacement therapy: scientific review. *Journal of the American Medical Association*, 2002, Vol. 288, Iss. 7, 872–881.

Rossouw, J. E., et al. Risks and benefits of estrogen plus progestin in healthy postmenopausal women: principal results from the Women's Health Initiative randomized controlled trial. *Journal of the American Medical Association*, 2002, Vol. 288, Iss. 3, 321–333.

Viscoli, C. M., et al. A clinical trial of estrogen-replacement therapy after ischemic stroke. *New England Journal of Medicine*, 2001, Vol. 345, Iss. 17, 1243–1249.

Vittinghoff, E., et al. Risk factors and secondary prevention in women with heart disease: the Heart and Estrogen/progestin Replacement Study. *Annals of Internal Medicine*, 2003, Vol. 138, Iss. 2, 81–89.

Chapter 4. Research and Emerging Therapies

Albert, M. A., et al. Effect of statin therapy on C-reactive protein levels: the pravastatin inflammation/CRP evaluation (PRINCE): a randomized trial and cohort study. *Journal of the American Medical Association*, 2001, Vol. 286, Iss. 1, 64–70.

Bartlett, C., J. Sterne, and M. Egger. What is newsworthy? Longitudinal study of the reporting of medical research in two British newspapers. *British Medical Journal*, 2002, Vol. 325, Iss. 7355, 81–84.

Collins, R. Heart protection study finds simvastatin reduces vascular risk in a wide range of high-risk patients. *American Journal of Managed Care*, 2002, Suppl., 6.

Freedman, S. B., and J. M. Isner. Therapeutic angiogenesis for coronary artery disease. *Annals of Internal Medicine*, 2002, Vol. 136, Iss. 1, 54–71.

Gregoratos, G., et al. ACC/AHA guidelines for implantation of cardiac pacemakers and antiarrhythmia devices: a report of the American College of Cardiology/American Heart Association Task Force on Practice Guidelines (Committee on Pacemaker Implantation). *Journal of the American College of Cardiology*, 1998, Vol. 31, Iss. 5, 1175–1209.

Grines, C. L., et al. Angiogenic Gene Therapy (AGENT) trial in patients with stable angina pectoris. *Circulation*, 2002, Vol. 105, Iss. 11, 1291–1297.

Herrington, D. M., et al. Statin therapy, cardiovascular events, and total mortality in the Heart and Estrogen/Progestin Replacement Study (HERS). *Circulation*, 2002, Vol. 105, Iss. 25, 2962–2967.

Jenkins, N. P., B. D. Prendergast, and M. Thomas. Drug eluting coronary stents. *British Medical Journal*, 2002, Vol. 325, Iss. 7376, 1315–1316.

Morice, M. C., et al. A randomized comparison of a sirolimus-eluting stent with a standard stent for coronary revascularization. *New England Journal of Medicine*, 2002, Vol. 346, Iss. 23, 1773–1780.

Moss. A. J., et al. Prophylactic implantation of a defibrillator in patients with myocardial infarction and reduced ejection fraction. *New England Journal of Medicine*, 2002, Vol. 346, Iss. 12, 877–883.

MRC/BHF Heart Protection Study of cholesterol lowering with simvastatin in 20,536 high-risk individuals: a randomised placebo-controlled trial. *Lancet*, 2002, Vol. 360, Iss. 9326, 7–22.

Pearson, T. A., et al. Markers of inflammation and cardiovascular disease: application to clinical and public health practice: a statement for healthcare professionals from the Centers for Disease Control and Prevention and the American Heart Association. *Circulation*, 2003, Vol. 107, Iss. 3, 499–511.

Ray, J. G., et al. Use of statins and the subsequent development of deep vein thrombosis. *Archives of Internal Medicine*, 2001, Vol. 161, Iss. 11, 1405–1410.

Ridker, P. M., et al. Comparison of C-reactive protein and low-density lipoprotein cholesterol levels in the prediction of first cardiovascular events. *New England Journal of Medicine*, 2002, Vol. 347, Iss. 20, 1557–1565.

Ross, R. Atherosclerosis—an inflammatory disease. *New England Journal of Medicine*, 1999, Vol. 340, Iss. 2, 115–126.

Waksman, R., et al. Use of localised intracoronary beta radiation in treatment of in-stent restenosis: the INHIBIT randomised controlled trial. *Lancet*, 2002, Vol. 359, Iss. 9306, 551–557.

Chapter 5. Staying Well and Prepared

Bridges, C. B., et al. Prevention and control of influenza. Recommendations of the Advisory Committee on Immunization Practices (ACIP). *Morbidity and Mortality Weekly Report*, 2002, Vol. 51, Iss. RR03, 1–31.

Bristow, M. R., et al. Cardiac-resynchronization therapy with or without an implantable defibrillator in advanced chronic heart failure. *New England Journal of Medicine*, 2002, Vol. 350, Iss. 21, 2140–2150.

Bush, D. E., et al. Even minimal symptoms of depression increase mortality risk after acute myocardial infarction. *American Journal of Cardiology*, 2001, Vol. 88, Iss. 4, 337–341.

Frasure-Smith, N., F. Lesperance, and M. Talajic. Depression following myocardial infarction. Impact on six-month survival. *Journal of the American Medical Association*, 1993, Vol. 270, Iss. 15, 1819–1825.

Glassman, A. H., and P. A. Shapiro. Depression and the course of coronary artery disease. *American Journal of Psychiatry*, 1998, Vol. 155, Iss. 1, 4–11.

Glassman, A. H., et al. Sertraline treatment of major depression in patients with acute MI or unstable angina. *Journal of the American Medical Association*, 2002, Vol. 288, Iss. 6, 701–709.

Guck, T. P., et al. Assessment and treatment of depression following myocardial infarction. *American Family Physician*, 2001, Vol. 64, Iss. 4, 641–648.

Keller, M. B., et al. A comparison of nefazodone, the cognitive behavioral-analysis system of psychotherapy, and their combination for the treatment of chronic depression. *New England Journal of Medicine*, 2000, Vol. 342, Iss. 20, 1462–1470.

Lavallee, P., et al. Association between influenza vaccination and reduced risk of brain infarction. *Stroke*, 2002, Vol. 33, Iss. 2, 513–518.

Mendes de Leon, C. F., et al. Depression and risk of coronary heart disease in elderly men and women: New Haven EPESE, 1982–1991. Established Populations for the Epidemiologic

Studies of the Elderly. *Archives of Internal Medicine*, 1998, Vol. 158, Iss. 21, 2341–2348.

Musselman, D. L., D. L. Evans, and C. B. Nemeroff. The relationship of depression to cardiovascular disease: epidemiology, biology, and treatment. *Archives of General Psychiatry*, 1998, Vol. 55, Iss. 7, 580–592.

Naghavi, M., et al. Association of influenza vaccination and reduced risk of recurrent myocardial infarction. *Circulation*, 2000, Vol. 102, Iss. 25, 3039–3045.

Nissen, S. E., et al. Effect of recombinant ApoA-I Milano on coronary atherosclerosis in patients with acute coronary syndromes: a randomized controlled trial. *Journal of the American Medical Association*, 2003, Vol. 290, Iss. 17, 2292–2300.

Penninx, B. W., et al. Depression and cardiac mortality: results from a community-based longitudinal study. *Archives of General Psychiatry*, 2001, Vol. 58, Iss. 3, 221–227.

Reynolds, C. F., 3rd, et al. Nortriptyline and interpersonal psychotherapy as maintenance therapies for recurrent major depression: a randomized controlled trial in patients older than 59 years. *Journal of the American Medical Association*, 1999, Vol. 281, Iss. 1, 39–45.

Rimm, E. B., et al. Moderate alcohol intake and lower risk of coronary heart disease: meta-analysis of effects on lipids and haemostatic factors. *British Medical Journal*, 1999, Vol. 319, Iss. 7224, 1523–1528.

Schulz, R., et al. Association between depression and mortality in older adults: the Cardiovascular Health Study. *Archives of Internal Medicine*, 2000, Vol. 160, Iss. 12, 1761–1768.

Thase, M. E., et al. Treatment of major depression with psychotherapy or psychotherapy-pharmacotherapy combinations. *Archives of General Psychiatry*, 1997, Vol. 54, Iss. 11, 1009–1015.

Appendices

Aggarwal, A., and P. A. Ades. Interactions of herbal remedies with prescription cardiovascular medications. *Coronary Artery Disease*, 2001, Vol. 12, Iss. 7, 581–584.

Ameer, B., and R. A. Weintraub. Drug interactions with grapefruit juice. *Clinical Pharmacokinetics*, 1997, Vol. 33, Iss. 2, 103–121.

Ament, P. W., J. G. Bertolino, and J. L. Liszewski. Clinically significant drug interactions. *American Family Physician*, 2000, Vol. 61, Iss. 6, 1745–1754.

Birkmeyer, J. D., et al. Hospital volume and surgical mortality in the United States. *New England Journal of Medicine*, 2002, Vol. 346, Iss. 15, 1128–1137.

Cheitlin, M. D., et al. ACC/AHA guidelines for the clinical application of echocardiography: executive summary. A report of the American College of Cardiology/American Heart Association Task Force on Practice Guidelines (Committee on Clinical Application of Echocardiography). Developed in collaboration with the American Society of Echocardiography. *Journal of the American College of Cardiology*, 1997, Vol. 29, Iss. 4, 862–879.

Crawford, M. H., et al. ACC/AHA guidelines for ambulatory electrocardiography: executive summary and recommendations. A report of the American College of Cardiology/American Heart Association Task Force on Practice Guidelines (Committee to Revise the Guidelines for Ambulatory Electrocardiography). *Circulation*, 1999, Vol. 100, Iss. 8, 886–893.

Eagle, K. A., et al. ACC/AHA guidelines for coronary artery bypass graft surgery: executive summary and recommendations. A report of the American College of Cardiology/American Heart Association Task Force on Practice Guidelines (Committee to Revise the 1991 Guidelines for Coronary Artery Bypass Graft Surgery). *Circulation*, 1999, Vol. 100, Iss. 13, 1464–1480.

Gibbons, R. J., et al. ACC/AHA guidelines for exercise testing: executive summary. A report of the American College of Cardiology/American Heart Association Task Force on Practice

Guidelines (Committee on Exercise Testing). *Circulation*, 1997, Vol. 96, Iss. 1, 345–354.

Hirshfeld, J.W., Jr., S.G. Ellis, and D.P. Faxon. Recommendations for the assessment and maintenance of proficiency in coronary interventional procedures: statement of the American College of Cardiology. *Journal of the American College of Cardiology*, 1998, Vol. 31, Iss. 3, 722–743.

Johnson, M.D., G. Newkirk, and J.R. White, Jr. Clinically significant drug interactions. *Postgraduate Medicine*, 1999, Vol. 105, Iss. 2, 193–195, 205–206.

Kane, G.C., and J.J. Lipsky. Drug-grapefruit juice interactions. *Mayo Clinic Proceedings*, 2000, Vol. 75, Iss. 9, 933–942.

O'Rourke, R.A., et al. American College of Cardiology/American Heart Association expert consensus document on electron-beam computed tomography for the diagnosis and prognosis of coronary artery disease. *Journal of the American College of Cardiology*, 2000, Vol. 36, Iss. 1, 326–340.

Ritchie, J.L., et al. Guidelines for clinical use of cardiac radionuclide imaging. Report of the American College of Cardiology/American Heart Association Task Force on Assessment of Diagnostic and Therapeutic Cardiovascular Procedures (Committee on Radionuclide Imaging), developed in collaboration with the American Society of Nuclear Cardiology. *Journal of the American College of Cardiology*, 1995, Vol. 25, Iss. 2, 521–547.

Scanlon, P.J., et al. ACC/AHA guidelines for coronary angiography: executive summary and recommendations. A report of the American College of Cardiology/American Heart Association Task Force on Practice Guidelines (Committee on Coronary Angiography) developed in collaboration with the Society for Cardiac Angiography and Interventions. *Circulation*, 1999, Vol. 99, Iss. 17, 2345–2357.

Schlant, R.C., et al. Guidelines for electrocardiography. A report of the American College of Cardiology/American Heart Association Task Force on Assessment of Diagnostic and Therapeutic Cardiovascular Procedures (Committee on Electrocardiography). *Circulation*, 1992, Vol. 85, Iss. 3, 1221–1228.

Smith, S. C., Jr., et al. ACC/AHA guidelines for percutaneous coronary intervention (revision of the 1993 PTCA guidelines)—executive summary. A report of the American College of Cardiology/American Heart Association Task Force on Practice Guidelines (Committee to Revise the 1993 Guidelines for Percutaneous Transluminal Coronary Angioplasty) endorsed by the Society for Cardiac Angiography and Interventions. *Circulation*, 2001, Vol. 103, Iss. 24, 3019–3041.

Smith, S. C., Jr., et al. AHA/ACC Scientific Statement: AHA/ACC guidelines for preventing heart attack and death in patients with atherosclerotic cardiovascular disease: 2001 update: a statement for healthcare professionals from the American Heart Association and the American College of Cardiology. *Circulation*, 2001, Vol. 104, Iss. 13, 1577–1579.

Spertus, J. A., et al. Development and evaluation of the Seattle Angina Questionnaire: a new functional status measure for coronary artery disease. Journal of the American College of Cardiology, 1995, Vol. 25, Iss. 2, 333–341.